THE CONCISE PERRIN TECHNIQUE

A handbook for patients

To Hilda and Bernard Perrin
... parents in a million

THE CONCISE PERRIN TECHNIQUE

A handbook for patients

A practical companion to
The Perrin Technique 2nd Edition

DR RAYMOND PERRIN

DO, PhD

Osteopath and Neuroscientist

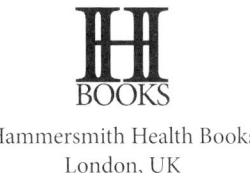

Hammersmith Health Books
London, UK

First published in 2021 by Hammersmith Health Books
– an imprint of Hammersmith Books Limited
4/4A Bloomsbury Square, London WC1A 2RP, UK
www.hammersmithbooks.co.uk

© 2021, Raymond Perrin

All rights reserved. No part of this publication may be reproduced, stored in any retrieval system or transmitted in any form or by any means, electronic, mechanical, photocopying, recording or otherwise, without the prior permission of the publishers and copyright holders.

The information contained in this book is for educational purposes only. It is the result of the study and the experience of the author. Whilst the information and advice offered are believed to be true and accurate at the time of going to press, neither the author nor the publisher can accept any legal responsibility or liability for any errors or omissions that may have been made or for any adverse effects which may occur as a result of following the recommendations given herein. Always consult a qualified medical practitioner if you have any concerns regarding your health.

British Library Cataloguing in Publication Data: A CIP record of this book is available from the British Library.

Print ISBN 978-1-78161-206-4
Ebook ISBN 978-1-78161-207-1

Commissioning editor: Georgina Bentliff
Designed and typeset by: Julie Bennett, Bespoke Publishing Ltd
Cover design by: Madeline Meckiffe
Index: Dr Laurence Errington
Production: Deborah Wehner of Moatvale Press, UK
Printed and bound by: TJ Books, Cornwall, UK
Images: page 84 top © Shutterstock/Tokarchuk Andrii; 84 bottom © Shutterstock/Sahara Prince; 85 top © Shutterstock/VagonPhoto; 85 bottom © Shutterstock/Shavlovskiy; page 86 © iStock bagi1998.

Contents

List of figures	ix
Acknowledgements	xii
About the author	xiii
Dear reader	1
Foreword: Jade Benson	3

Chapter 1: The basics: How the Perrin Technique works	**7**
The Perrin Technique: the facts	8
Fact 1: Fluid flow	8
Fact 2: Getting the toxins out	9
Fact 3: The pumping mechanism	10
Fact 4: The sympathetic nervous system	11
Fact 5: Biofeedback	11
Fact 6: What goes wrong	12
Fact 7: Build-up of toxins	13
Conclusion	15

Chapter 2: ME/CFS and FMS: What's really going on?	**17**
Blackout	18
ME/CFS: 'The black hole of medicine'	19
The naming of the disease	20
Defining ME/CFS	21
Fibromyalgia	22
Conclusion	23

Chapter 3: The role of toxins in ME/CFS and FMS	**25**
Pollutants	25
Effects of neurotoxins	27
Diet and toxicity	28
Predisposition to toxicity	29
Conclusion	30

Chapter 4: The stages leading to ME/CFS and FMS	31
The physical signs of ME/CFS and FMS	33
1. Longstanding thoracic spinal problems	36
2. Varicose lymphatics and 3. Perrin's Point	38
4. Tenderness at the coeliac or solar plexus	43
5. Disturbance in the cranio-sacral rhythm	44
The two minor physical signs	45
Scoring the patient	46
Conclusion	48

Chapter 5: Treatment using the Perrin Technique	49
The magic bullet?	49
How osteopathy helps	52
Lubrication for effleurage	53
The concertina and siphon effects	53
Reducing inflammation	54
Perrin Technique protocol for FMS	55
Post-traumatic FMS	56
The 10 steps of the Perrin Technique	57
After treatment	59
Self-help advice	59
Dorsal rotation and shrugging exercises	61
Cross-crawl	64
Strengthening exercises for hypermobile spinal joints	64
Hypermobility of the lower lumbar region	68
Home-massage routine	68
Nasal release	69
Facial massage	69
Head massage	70
Self-massage to front of neck	71
Breast massage	72
Back massage	73
Back of neck massage	73
Full routine	73
Active head rest	75

Returning to good health	76
Diet and nutrition	77
Supplements	78
Getting worse before getting better	81
The jigsaw puzzle analogy	83
For colds and flu	86
Frequency of treatment	88
Conclusion	89
Case: Noel's story	90
Appendix 1: Frequently asked questions	**93**
What are the causes of ME/CFS and FMS?	93
What symptoms can you get with ME/CFS and FMS?	95
Is fibromyalgia syndrome (FMS) a different disease to ME/CFS?	101
Who suffers from ME/CFS and FMS?	102
What does the Perrin Technique treatment involve?	103
What responses to treatment should I expect?	104
How quickly will I recover?	105
How often should I receive the Perrin Technique treatment?	105
What are the dos and don'ts for patients with ME/CFS and FMS?	106
How much exercise and activity can I do?	113
What hobbies can I do safely?	116
Is technology safe to use?	116
When can I return to work/education?	117
Are there any dos and don'ts on commuting?	118
If I am improving, can I go on holiday?	119
Is it safe to get pregnant with ME/CFS or FMS?	120
If I require surgery, what precautions are needed?	121
How important are environmental factors?	122
Can the Perrin Technique help with other conditions?	124
Once I have recovered, can the illness recur?	126

>   Can ME/CFS and FMS be prevented? 127

Appendix 2: Common pathological and radiological tests 129
Appendix 3: The Perrin Questionnaire for chronic fatigue syndrome/ME (PQ-CFS) 141
Appendix 4: Useful names and addresses 146

Afterword: Aisling Wharton 158
Index 160

List of figures

Fig. 1   Jade at home before starting the Perrin Technique, desperately ill, housebound for many years, wheelchair-bound for two years, being cared for by her devoted mother, Barbara Hodgkinson.   4

Fig. 2   Jade well enough after 18 months of treatment to climb with her parents Barbara and Andrew, and myself, plus a group of friends (not pictured) to the top of the highest mountain in England, Scafell Pike, to raise funds for my research.   5

Fig. 3   Former severe ME/CFS patients Jade Benson and Jen Turner at Jade's wedding.   6

Fig. 4   The thoracic duct (the central lymphatic drainage system into the blood).   10

Fig. 5   Restricted drainage of toxins from the central nervous system.   14

Fig. 6   The downward spiral into ME/CFS.   14

Fig. 7   The main feature of fibromyalgia is pain in the four quadrants of the body.   23

Fig 8.   The observed physical signs of ME/CFS.   36

Fig. 9   Comparative photographs showing a flattened mid-thoracic spine. Photo (a) shows the familiar flattening of the mid-thoracic spine seen in many ME/CFS and FMS patients. This differs from a normal spinal posture in the healthy subject, photo (b).   38

Fig.10   Examining a male patient for 'Perrin's Point'. Gentle pressure at a point slightly superior and lateral to the left nipple, 'Perrin's Point'(X). The amount of sensitivity at this point appears to correspond to the severity of lymphatic

	engorgement in the breast tissue and also seems to mirror the gravity of the other symptoms.	39
Fig. 11	Schematic illustration showing normal flow within a healthy lymphatic vessel. The valves in this healthy vessel are intact, preventing any backflow, thus maintaining a healthy, unidirectional drainage (note the smooth muscular wall of the lymphangion regulated by sympathetic nerves).	41
Fig. 12.	The development of varicose megalymphatics: (a) The normal lymph flow before the illness. (b) Reversal of the central lymphatic pump forces the colourless lymph fluid back, damaging the valves that separate the adjacent collecting vessels (lymphangia). (c) The lymphangia expand due to the pressure and volume of the backward flowing lymph. This leads to the large beaded vessels (varicose mega-lymphatics) palpated (felt with the fingertips) just beneath the skin in the chest of ME/CFS and FMS patients.	42
Fig. 13	Right subclavicular varicose megalymphatics, lacking the bluish hue of varicose veins, in patient with ME/CFS (see colour plate 4 in second edition).	43
Fig. 14	Upper thoracic rotation exercise.	61
Fig. 15	Mid-thoracic rotation exercise.	62
Fig. 16	Lower thoracic rotation exercise.	63
Fig. 17	Shoulder rolling exercise.	63
Fig. 18	Cervical isometrics: (a) Attempting to bend head forward, prevented by gentle backwards pressure of hands. (b) Attempting to bend head back, prevented by gentle forward pressure of hands.	66
Fig. 19	Cervical isometrics: (a) Attempting to bend head to the left, prevented by gentle counter-pressure of left hand. (b) Attempting to bend head to the right, prevented by gentle counter-pressure of right hand.	66

List of Figures

Fig. 20	Cervical isometrics: (a) Attempting to tuck in chin, prevented by gentle forward counter-pressure of thumbs. (b) Attempting to push chin forward, prevented by gentle backwards counter-pressure of fingers.	67
Fig. 21	Nasal release.	69
Fig. 22	Facial self-massage.	70
Fig. 23	Self-massage to head.	71
Fig. 24	Self-massage to front of neck.	71
Fig. 25	Self-massage of the breast.	72
Fig. 26	Head rest exercise.	76
Fig. 27	An ME/CFS patient and her daily medication.	79
Fig. 28	The same patient after receiving the Perrin Technique and reducing her supplements and medication intake.	80
Fig. 29	Simple jigsaw puzzle of a few pieces, which is easy to solve.	84
Fig. 30	Complex jigsaw puzzle with lots of sea and sky, making it very difficult to solve without the guidance of the corners and edges.	84
Fig. 31	A random approach to solving a jigsaw puzzle, without any clues.	85
Fig. 32	An overwhelmingly complicated jigsaw puzzle representing a really complex case of ME/CFS or FMS.	85
Fig. 33	Completing the puzzle with the corners and edges in place first.	86
Fig. 34	Adapted back sculling technique.	114

Acknowledgements

Gratitude is a vaccine, an antitoxin, and an antiseptic.
John Henry Jowett, British preacher 1864-1923

Thanks to my colleagues and all the amazing patients, plus their families and friends, who over the years have increased awareness of my work and raised most of the funds for my continued research. There have been so many kind donations and hundreds of wonderful people who have organised dinners, dances and musical evenings, jogged hundreds of miles, climbed mountains, cycled in cartoon outfits, walked in deep-sea diver suits, swum lakes and kayaked down mountain rivers, all to help pay the costs for the ongoing scientific studies that are needed to further understand how the Perrin Technique can help the millions of sufferers of ME/CFS, fibromyalgia and now long-COVID.

A special mention for the fund-raising efforts of Perrin Technique practitioner Sue Capstick and her team of physiotherapists, friends and family who annually take part and offer treatments for the runners in the Wigan 10K event, plus the past and present trustees of the Fund for Osteopathic Research into ME (FORME Trust) for all their continuous help and support.

Ray Perrin, March 2021

About the author

Raymond N Perrin DO PhD is a Registered Osteopath and Neuroscientist specialising in myalgic encephalomyelitis/chronic fatigue syndrome (ME/CFS). His present academic posts include Honorary Clinical Research Fellow at the School of Health Sciences in the Faculty of Biology, Medicine and Health at the University of Manchester, Manchester, UK and Honorary Senior Lecturer in the Allied Health Professions Research Unit, University of Central Lancashire, Preston, UK. He is also Research Director of the FORME Trust and Founder and Clinical Director of the Perrin Clinic™.

Treating a patient for backpain in 1989 led him to the concept that there was a structural basis to ME/CFS. He has spent over 30 years conducting clinical trials, researching the medical facts and sifting the scientific evidence while successfully treating an increasing number of ME/CFS and fibromyalgia sufferers and teaching fellow osteopaths, chiropractors and physiotherapists the fundamentals of the Perrin Technique.

For his service to osteopathy, Dr Perrin was appointed a vice-patron of the University College of Osteopathy (formerly the BSO) and in 2015 became the very first winner of the Research and Practice Award from the Institute of Osteopathy.

Dear reader,

This is a patient handbook and companion volume to the second edition of my book *The Perrin Technique: How to diagnose and treat chronic fatigue syndrome/ME and fibromyalgia via the lymphatic drainage of the brain*.

The first edition, *The Perrin Technique: How to beat chronic fatigue syndrome/ME*, was published in 2007 and was based on my doctorate, which I received after 11 years of research into myalgic encephalomyelitis at the University of Salford, UK.

Since 2007, I have continued my research and have been kept busy lecturing to the medical and scientific world on the lymphatic system of the brain and how it is disturbed in ME/CFS and fibromyalgia, plus teaching my techniques to those who wish to learn my approach. However, it wasn't easy in the beginning, as there was no proof that a lymphatic system of the brain even existed in the first place, never mind any problems with its drainage.

Everything changed in 2012, when there was a breakthrough discovery at the University of Rochester in New York State. Scientists, using a new type of brain scan, were able visually to show that the fluid in the brain did indeed drain into the lymphatics, and in 2015 a group from the University of Virginia discovered true lymphatic vessels lining the brain in mice. Finally, after so many years, the foundation of my main theory as to what was going wrong in patients with ME/CFS was being backed up by scientific discovery…albeit in rodents. It was then that I started writing the second edition of my book and during this time, further scans of human brains have revealed a major system of lymphatic drainage of the central nervous system which may, according to scientists around the world, provide a pathway that is affected in many neurological disorders. I developed the Perrin Technique in 1989 to improve this drainage system, so it is nice to know that finally science has caught up.

My publisher, Georgina, instructed me to just start writing and let her know when I was finished. Well, after over five years, the second edition has finally been completed with over 500 pages containing all the facts a patient, practitioner and/or scientist needs to know about ME/CFS and fibromyalgia syndrome (FMS). I have added FMS to the second edition as it is very similar, and has, in my opinion, the same causal factors as ME/CFS, plus my treatment has helped patients with both conditions for over 30 years.

If you have ME/CFS or FMS and are unable to concentrate on long text, or wish/ have to save the cost of the much larger version, this handbook is for you. It sums up my theory of diagnosis and treatment of these complex diseases, including the Perrin Technique treatment plan. This will hopefully guide you, the patient, along your own individual road to recovery. I endeavour to keep the explanations as simple as possible in this companion handbook as the comprehensive book can provide all the extra detail you might want. If, after reading this, you wish to fully understand the complexities of diagnosis and treatment of ME/CFS and FMS and related conditions, complete with hundreds of scientific references, the second edition is waiting to be read.

If you wish to start the Perrin Technique, please try to find a practitioner near to you who is a trained and a licensed Perrin Technique practitioner if possible. If there are none in your neighbourhood, seek out a practitioner trained and experienced in both cranial techniques and manual therapy but preferably an osteopath, physiotherapist/physical therapist or chiropractor. They will be able to understand the detailed second edition, which contains a comprehensive section on other clinical conditions that could cause fatigue and diseases that commonly occur in patients with ME/CFS and FMS.

Once the practitioner has read the second edition of *The Perrin Technique*, they should be able to follow the instructions and be equipped to help you. It is better not to rely just on the self-massage and exercises in this handbook though it is very important that you do these as they will help. It is always best to do the whole treatment programme under the direction of a qualified practitioner to confirm the diagnosis and to improve your outlook.

If your condition is more complicated, the second edition contains advice that will guide you, the patient, and your practitioner to help in even the most complex presentations that could occur together with ME/CFS and FMS.

I wish you every success with your treatment and progress to better health.

Raymond Perrin, January 2021

Foreword

Jade Benson: recovered ME/CFS patient

I developed ME after a nasty bout of glandular fever at age 6. I was eventually diagnosed after my first 'crash' at 11 years old, shortly after starting secondary school. Over the next seven years my condition got progressively worse, seeing many 'crashes' and meaning that I couldn't be educated in mainstream school because of the severity of my condition. By the time I reached my 18th birthday, I was extremely unwell.

I was wheelchair-bound, unable to stand for more than a few seconds, light sensitive, noise sensitive, very nauseous and in constant severe pain and fatigue. After so many years of being severely ill my body was giving up, and at 18, so was I. I had to rely on my parents as carers, couldn't leave the house and had no quality of life, with no end in sight.

We heard about the Perrin Technique from a family friend who also had ME. Her mum had been told about the treatment by a hospital nurse whilst receiving treatment for cancer, and my friend thought the information was worth passing on. As I was too unwell, my mum did some research on the Perrin Technique and agreed it was worth a go.

Until this point no other treatment had helped me, including seven years under a paediatric consultant, a referral to the head of paediatric ME for the country, graded exercise, pacing, allergy testing, diets and several alternative therapies. We felt that this was my last chance to get better as I was deteriorating every week (see Figure 1).

We met with Dr Perrin on 17th February 2010 and he, and the treatment, made immediate sense to us. He explained ME in a way nobody else ever had; all the symptoms that other doctors had brushed off, looked confused at, or had made me feel like they were 'all in my head' suddenly had a real medical explanation, and – thankfully – an answer. I was examined by Dr Perrin and officially and positively diagnosed with ME. I was graded at 2/10 on the Perrin

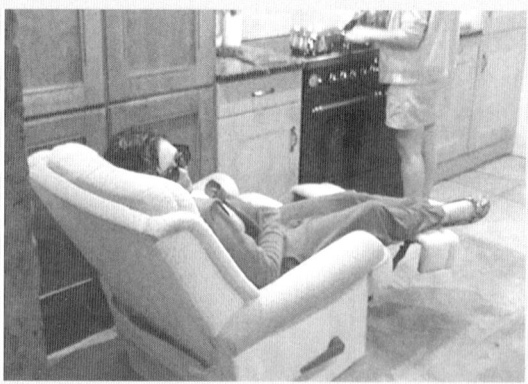

Fig. 1 Jade at home before starting the Perrin Technique, desperately ill, housebound for many years, wheelchair-bound for two years, being cared for by her devoted mother, Barbara Hodgkinson.

scale, which is severe, but I was still able to be helped. I came away from the clinic feeling hopeful for the first time in many years. I knew I had a long way to go but was stubbornly determined that I could get there. I started a programme of treatment soon after, with my weekly treatment being done in nearby Longridge and overseen by Dr Perrin due to my severity.

As expected, I got worse before I got better, and my condition deteriorated quickly. After one particular treatment with Dr Perrin in around April 2010, I reacted very severely and was partially paralysed for 24 hours. This reaction, although rare and frightening at the time, was the best thing that could have happened to me as once I had got through it, my recovery accelerated and I was soon seeing vast improvements in my condition. I took my first steps shortly after this reaction and dumped the wheelchair for good in June 2010, a mere four and a half months after starting my Perrin journey. By September, I was working part-time, had enrolled in college, and was practising for my driving test which I passed the next month. I was starting to finally lead a normal life for the first time in 11 years.

A year after I had ditched the wheelchair, I challenged myself and did a sponsored climb up Scafell Pike, the tallest peak in England, in aid of the charity which backs the Perrin Technique, accompanied by Dr Perrin, my parents and several friends (see Figure 2). On reaching the top and looking out over the Lake District I knew I had done it and my life would never be the same. I was never going back to being that ill shell of a person thanks to Dr Perrin and the Perrin Technique.

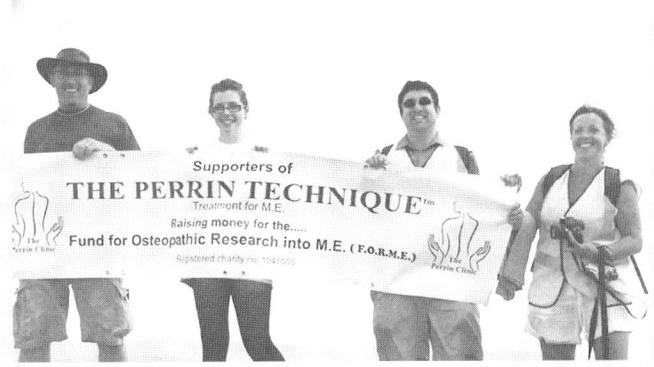

Fig. 2 Jade well enough after 18 months of treatment to climb with her parents Barbara and Andrew, and myself, plus a group of friends (not pictured) to the top of the highest mountain in England, Scafell Pike, to raise funds for my research.

Nine years on and, although I still have treatment every couple of months to ensure I stay well, I am largely symptom free. I am now married (see Figure 3), have a 3-year-old son and am expecting my second child. I have a normal, happy, healthy life now. Without the treatment, there's no way I would have the life I have today, and I am forever grateful for the second chance at life that it gave me.

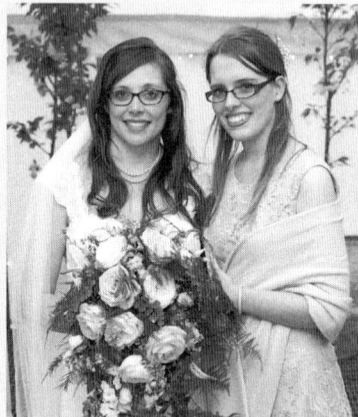

Fig. 3 Former severe ME/CFS patients Jade Benson and Jen Turner at Jade's wedding.

Jade Benson, Lancashire, UK

Chapter 1

The basics: How the Perrin Technique works

My theory for the diagnosis and treatment of ME/CFS started with one patient: this case was the first and perhaps the most dramatic of all the ME/CFS patients I have treated. In 1989 an executive, who shall be referred to as Mr E, walked into my city-centre practice, in Manchester, where I ran a clinic specialising in treating sports injuries. He had been a top cyclist, racing for one of the premier teams in the north-west of England. He had suffered from a recurring, low back pain, which, after examination, I had diagnosed to be a strain of the pelvic joints.

While treating his pelvis, I noted that the upper part of his back was particularly restricted. I enquired whether or not he had any prior problems in his upper back, and he acknowledged that for years, during his cycling, he had experienced a dull ache across his shoulders and at the top of his back. This in itself was nothing significant, as it was very common to find cyclists with pelvic problems and a stiff and disturbed curvature in the thoracic spine (the upper part of the backbone between the waist and the neck). What was interesting was the fact that, for the past seven years, Mr E had been diagnosed with ME/CFS. He complained of tingling in both hands and a 'muzzy' feeling in his head. He suffered general fatigue and an ache in his knees, as well as the pain in his back and shoulders. He had been forced to stop racing since the onset of the disorder. This patient was one of many who came to me after being diagnosed by their doctor, or specialist, as suffering from ME/CFS.

As I have said, he originally attended for treatment to his lower back. At that time, although I had helped other patients with ME/CFS, I had done no research into the disease, and I had no specific treatment programme for the disorder. With only five treatments, Mr E's back was better, but, most incredibly, the signs and symptoms of ME/CFS had drastically improved. He was symptom-free after a mere two months from the start of treatment. After many years he continued to remain healthy and the last news I heard of him was that he had moved to Holland, cycling with the same power and zeal that he had used to enjoy prior to his illness.

It was after helping this patient that I realised that there must be a correlation between the mechanical strain on the thoracic spine and ME/CFS. Although I had not set out to help the fatigue signs and symptoms in this patient, I had done exactly that by improving his posture and increasing movement in his spine. My thoughts turned to the other ME/CFS patients that I had treated for back pain and biomechanical strain. The restriction of the dorsal spine was a common factor that could not be ignored. Since 1989, thousands of patients with signs and symptoms of ME/CFS have visited my clinic and also practices all over the world run by practitioners trained in the Perrin Technique. None of them has presented with exactly the same symptoms but all have shared common structural and physical signs. This cannot be dismissed purely as coincidence. So, what is really going on?

The Perrin Technique: the facts

Fact 1: Fluid flow

A fluid flows around the brain and continues up and down the spinal cord: this is the cerebrospinal fluid. This fluid has many functions – for example, as a protective buffer to the central nervous system and for supplying nutrients to the brain. However, one function has been discussed in osteopathic medicine since the 1860s but has received significant scientific attention only in recent years and that is the role it plays in the drainage of large molecules.

In fact, not only is there visual evidence of the drainage system detailed in the first edition of my book, but actual lymphatic vessels have since been discovered in the membranes of the brain in both animal and human studies.

Fact 2: Getting the toxins out

The lymphatic system is an organisation of tubes around the body that provides a drainage system secondary to the blood flow. Why does the body need a secondary system to cope with poisons or foreign bodies in the tissues? Are the veins not good enough? The answer in one important word is 'size'. The blood does process poisons and particles, which enter the blood circulatory system via the walls of the microscopic blood vessels known as the capillaries. Their walls resemble a fine mesh which acts as a filter, thus allowing only small molecules to enter the bloodstream itself. When the blood reaches the liver, detoxification takes place, cleansing the blood of its impurities.

Larger molecules of toxins often need breaking down before entering the blood circulation, and they begin this process of detoxification in the lymph nodes on the way to drainage points just below the collar bone into two large veins (the subclavian veins), with most of the body's lymph draining into the left subclavian vein (see Figure 4).

The capillary beds of lymphatic vessels, known as 'terminal' or 'initial lymphatics', take in any size of molecule via a wall that resembles the gill of a fish, opening as wide as is necessary to engulf the foreign body. The lymphatics also help to dispose of some toxins and impurities through the skin (via perspiration), urine, bowel movements and our breath. Once toxins have drained into the subclavian veins, they eventually find their way into the liver and, as is the case with normal circulatory toxins, are broken down by the liver.

The Perrin Technique

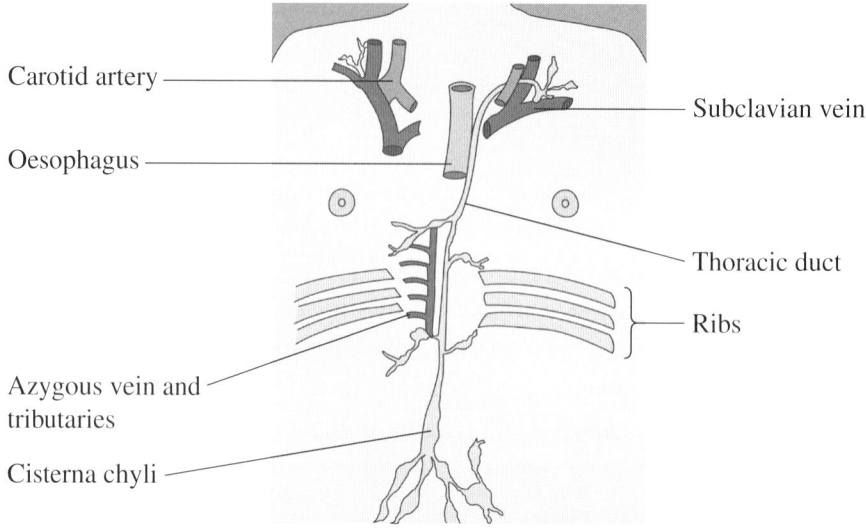

Fig. 4 The thoracic duct (the central lymphatic drainage system into the blood).

Fact 3: The pumping mechanism

For over 300 years, from 1622 when Italian physician and anatomist Gasparo (Gaspere) Aselli (1581 – 1626) discovered the lymphatic system, it was thought not to have a pump of its own. Its flow was believed to depend on the massaging effect of the surrounding muscles and the blood vessels lying next to the lymphatics, akin to squeezing toothpaste up the tube. However, we now know that the collecting vessels and ducts of the lymphatic system have smooth muscle walls, and Professor John Kinmonth, a London chest surgeon, discovered in the 1960s that the main drainage of the lymphatics, the thoracic duct, has a major pumping mechanism in its walls and that this is controlled by the sympathetic nervous system. If there is a disturbance of the sympathetic nervous system, the thoracic duct pumping mechanism may push the lymph fluid in the wrong direction and lead to a further build-up of toxins in the body.

Chapter 1

Fact 4: The sympathetic nervous system

The sympathetic nervous system is part of the autonomic nervous system, which deals with all the automatic functions of the body. Although it is known for being the system which helps us in times of danger and stress, often referred to as the 'fight or flight' system, the sympathetic nervous system is also important in controlling blood flow and the normal functioning of all the organs of the body, such as the heart, the kidneys and the bowel. We know it is vital for healthy lymphatic drainage. In ME/CFS and FMS sufferers, the sympathetic nervous system will have been placed under stress for many years before the onset of the signs and symptoms. This stress may be of a physical nature due to postural strain or an old injury, or it may be emotional stress, or environmental, such as pollution, or due to stress on the immune system due to infection or allergy.

The sympathetic nerves spread out from the thoracic spine to all parts of the body. The hypothalamus, just above the brain stem, acts as an integrator for autonomic functions, receiving regulatory input from other regions of the brain, especially the limbic system which involves emotion, motivation, learning and memory. Significantly, the hypothalamus also controls all the hormones of the body.

Fact 5: Biofeedback

The hypothalamus controls hormones by a process called biofeedback. This mechanism can be explained with the following example. If the sugar levels in the body are too low, it may be due to a rise in the hormone insulin, which is produced in the pancreas, which lies in the upper right side of the abdomen beneath the liver. Insulin, like other hormones, is a large protein molecule that travels through the blood and stimulates the breakdown of sugar. It passes from the blood into the hypothalamus, which will calculate if more or less insulin production is required and, accordingly, send a message to the pancreas to make the necessary adjustments.

The region of the hypothalamus is one of a few sections of the brain that allow the transfer of large molecules into the brain from the blood. In all other parts of the brain there is a filter known as the blood–brain barrier (BBB) allowing only small molecules to pass into the brain.

Unfortunately in many disease states, a damaged or disturbed BBB means that further large toxic molecules can invade the brain and wreak havoc on the normal functioning of the central nervous system, and in ME/CFS it has now been proven that many immune cells that promote inflammation do just that.

Fact 6: What goes wrong

The central nervous system, composed of the brain and the spinal cord, is the only region in the body that for hundreds of years was believed to have no true lymphatic system. Since we now know the lymphatics exist to drain large molecules, what can the central nervous system do if attacked by large toxins? It has now been demonstrated that the cerebrospinal fluid (see Fact 1) drains toxins along minute gaps next to blood vessels and then into the lymphatic system outside the head through perforations in the skull. The lymphatic vessels found in the head and around the spine take the toxins away via the thoracic duct and right lymphatic duct (see Figure 4) into the blood and the liver where they are broken down.

This drainage mechanism has now been filmed, with the largest amount draining through a bony plate (the cribriform plate) situated above the nose. The toxins then drain into lymphatic vessels in the tissue around the nasal sinuses. There is further drainage down similar channels next to blood vessels supplying other cranial nerves, especially the ones in the eye, ear and cheek respectively, and also down the spinal cord outwards to pockets of lymphatic vessels running alongside the spine.

The neuro-lymphatic drainage has been shown to occur during deep restorative sleep known as delta-wave sleep. Most patients with ME/CFS and FMS complain that they don't get enough sleep and that, when they do, they still feel exhausted. The problem for them is that though they may often have plenty of sleep, it isn't the restorative kind as it is consists of a high proportion of shallow, non-restorative alpha-waves.

Researchers at Stanford University in the USA have shown that ME/CFS patients have fewer delta-waves during the night, but too many during the day. The drainage of the brain and spinal cord occurs more during waking hours in ME/CFS and FMS, making those patients feel ill and shattered during the daytime. However, during the night in ME/CFS and FMS, the brain switches on, leading to the 'wired and fired' state, affecting most patients' ability to fall asleep.

Not only does the type of sleep affect neuro-lymphatic drainage, but it is the position a person adopts during sleep that is also vitally important. A side-lying posture during sleep aids neuro-lymphatic drainage as well as being the best position for the spine in general. Often, I am asked, 'Which side is best?' With regard to neuro-lymphatic drainage, I don't think it matters that much and I would advise you to start with lying on the side you feel most comfortable on. However, the left side is believed to be the better for improving venous return to the heart and also has been shown to reduce heartburn.

To maintain a balanced spine in bed, as well as lying on your side, I recommend a small pillow, such as a scatter cushion, placed between your knees throughout the night.

Fact 7: Build-up of toxins

In ME/CFS, I believe it is these drainage pathways, in both the head and the spine, that are not working sufficiently, leading to a build-up of toxins within the central nervous system. The reasons for drainage problems can vary from patient to patient. It may be trauma to the head from an accident; it may be hereditary or due to a problem at birth. The spine may become out of alignment – especially in very active teenagers – which can lead to a disturbance in the normal drainage (see Figure 5). If the spine and brain are both affected, the increased toxicity will disturb hypothalamic function and thus will further affect sympathetic control of the central lymphatic vessels. This in turn pumps more toxins back into the tissues and the brain, causing a vicious circle to ensue (see Figure 6).

The Perrin Technique

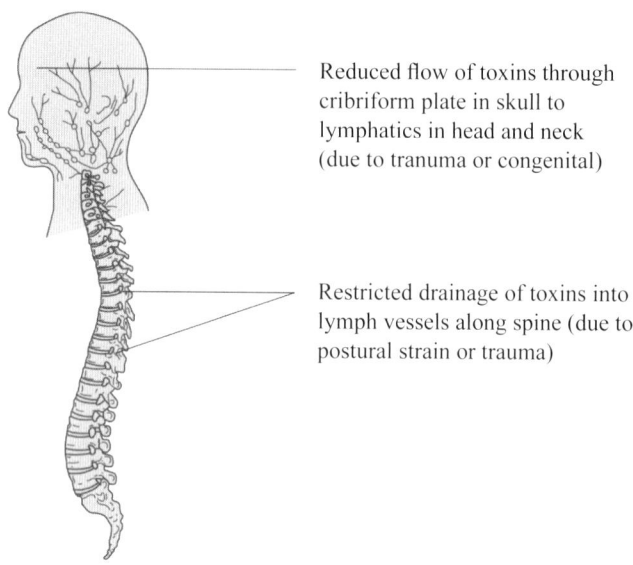

Fig. 5 Restricted drainage of toxins from the central nervous system.

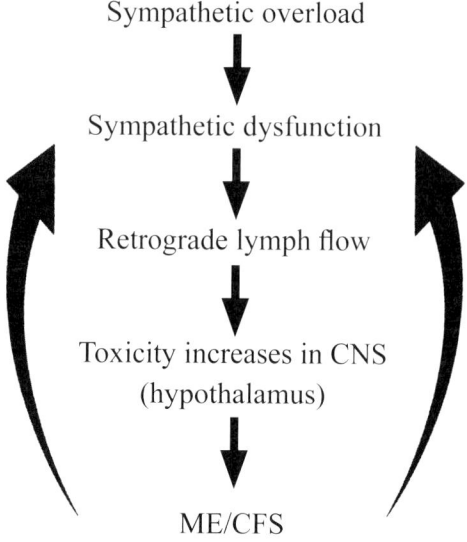

Fig. 6 The downward spiral into ME/CFS.

Chapter 1

This vicious circle results in the symptoms I describe in detail in Chapter 4, including varicose lymphatics, specific tender points especially 'Perrin's Point', and tenderness of the solar plexus (see pages 33-46) – symptoms that I have found in almost all ME/CFS patients in my 30+ year practice. It also can result in a varied assortment of additional symptoms that are often dismissed by healthcare professionals as unrelated because the underlying mechanism that unites them is not understood. These over 100 symptoms are listed in Appendix 1 (page 93) and explained in detail in *The Perrin Technique 2nd Edition*.

Conclusion

ME/CFS is very much a biomechanical disorder with clear and diagnosable physical signs, including disturbed spinal posture, varicose enlarged lymph vessels and specific tender points related to sympathetic nerve disturbance and backflow of lymphatic fluid. The fluid drainage from the brain to the lymphatics moves in a rhythm that can be palpated (felt with the fingertips) using cranial osteopathic techniques. A trained practitioner can feel a disturbance of the cranial rhythm in ME/CFS sufferers.

The Perrin Technique helps drain the toxins away from the central nervous system and incorporates manual techniques that stimulate the healthy flow of lymphatic and cerebrospinal fluid and improve spinal mechanics. This in turn reduces the toxic overload to the central nervous system which subsequently reduces the strain on the sympathetic nervous system, and this ultimately aids a return to good health.

Chapter 2

ME/CFS and FMS: What's really going on?

Chronic fatigue syndrome affects the communication between the internal organs and the musculoskeletal components of the body. This organ of communication is known as the **sympathetic nervous system** which may be likened to a transmission station in a power grid.

In our homes and at work, we use electricity for lighting, cooking, refrigerating and freezing, for electrical appliances, and for music centres, TVs and computers. The electrical energy required is produced by power stations and is monitored by controllers in transmission stations, which channel the amount of electricity through to us, the consumers.

If we were all suddenly to use substantially more electricity, simultaneously, the transmission station would allow more electricity to flow, signalling to the power stations to produce more energy. This occurs, for example, at half-time during major international televised sporting events, when everybody turns on the kettle at the same time to make a cup of tea.

If something were to go wrong with the operator, or the equipment in the transmission station were to develop a fault, the power required to cope with the increased demand would be insufficient. This would eventually lead to a power cut and blackout. Alternatively, if a situation were to arise when too much electricity passed into the household's supply, an overload or power surge could damage the appliances in use at that time.

In the body, the brain and the muscles are the principal 'electrical appliances', utilising most of the energy produced. The power station of the body is the gastrointestinal system (gut), together with the respiratory system, which consumes fuel in the form of food together with oxygen to produce the energy.

The sympathetic nervous system is the transmission station, which connects the visceral 'power station' of the body to the musculoskeletal 'appliance'.

Blackout

When we are active, the sympathetic nervous system stimulates an increase of energy production and a release of stored energy. If this is not accomplished, the result is that the muscles will not receive the nutrients normally obtained from the blood, and the natural function of the muscles, nerves and joints will break down. There will be a power cut in our body and we will suffer fatigue.

This is precisely what occurs in patients suffering from ME/CFS. The body demands more energy, especially when under any form of stress, mental or physical. However, the mechanism normally operated to transform the stored energy into a usable form is not functioning, and thus the patient's body simply stops working effectively.

It is therefore not surprising that ME/CFS is a profoundly debilitating disorder and requires as much rest as possible to reverse the process by minimising the amount of stress on the body. The power station analogy explains why some sufferers seem to display signs of too much sympathetic activity, such as palpitations and excessive sweating, as well as reduced sympathetic activity, such as fatigue and low blood pressure. The fault with the 'transmission station' could lead to the body working in overdrive as well as the power cut scenario, and sometimes in the same patient at the same time. Reducing the demand on the sympathetic nervous system helps the patient onto the road to a full recovery.

Chapter 2

ME/CFS: 'The black hole of medicine'

ME/CFS has been given more names than probably any other disease, and yet there is still no universally accepted way of positively diagnosing it, and therefore, treatment remains controversial and, by many schools of thought, unscientific. Because the disease is such an enigma, with so many problems affecting the patients and countless different ideas being bandied about as to the cause, it is often diagnosed without practitioners following the basic and essential procedure in clinical medicine – namely, that of properly examining the patient before making a diagnosis or providing treatment. As it is often diagnosed when other, more common conditions have been excluded, it has been called 'The black hole of medicine'.

Many patients who suffer from ME/CFS are left untreated, with the physician hoping that the patient will spontaneously recover, learn to live with the problem, or change doctors. Despite the fact that the World Health Organization (WHO) has recognised myalgic encephalomyelitis (ME) as a neurological disease since at least 1969, when it published the 8th edition of *The International Statistical Classification of Diseases and Related Health Problems* (ICD-8), and despite thousands of scientific papers being published which demonstrate that ME/CFS is a real physical disease, with many different pathological findings, there are still many GPs who refuse to believe in a physical source of the symptoms and refer their patients to a psychiatrist. Meanwhile, the WHO continues in the 10th edition to classify ME/CFS as a disease of the nervous system (ICD-10 G93.3).

Diagnosis of many conditions employs techniques such as MRI (magnetic resonance imaging), using computer-enhanced prints of the body. Electron microscopy shows each cell of the body in greater detail than ever before. Endless numbers of viruses have been identified, and yet, there are still some common ailments that continue to baffle medical scientists, including ME/CFS and fibromyalgia; slowly, however, more and more members of the scientific and medical community are beginning to understand these diseases.

The naming of the disease

Fibromyalgia or fibromyalgia syndrome (FMS), has not suffered as much from an identity crisis as has ME/CFS. FMS is now accepted worldwide as a rheumatological disease affecting the musculo-skeletal system and causing widespread pain.

This acceptance is completely different from the way the medical and scientific camps have viewed the disorder known to many as ME or chronic fatigue syndrome (or post-viral fatigue syndrome, or post-infectious disease syndrome, or chronic Epstein-Barr syndrome, etc, etc). In the United States it used to be commonly referred to as chronic fatigue and immune dysfunction syndrome (CFIDS). It has been known by so many names that eminent American specialist Dr David Bell referred to it as the 'disease of a thousand names' in his seminal work.

Most diseases are classified according to the type of change that takes place in the cells of the body – e.g. chronic lymphocytic leukaemia. Some diseases are categorised according to causative factors – e.g. TB caused by *Mycobacterium tuberculosis* or COVID-19. The problem with chronic fatigue syndrome (ME/CFS) is that it does not fit into any particular category; it is so diverse in its signs and symptoms that no specific disease classification fits the bill. There are, however, five key signs that I find in almost all patients (see page 36) and then a plethora of additional, seemingly unrelated symptoms that I have included in the Appendix (page 93); their relationship to underlying problems with lymphatic drainage and the dysfunctional sympathetic nervous system are described in detail in *The Perrin Technique 2nd Edition*. Thus, we have the term 'myalgic encephalomyelitis' (ME): myalgic refers to pain in muscles and encephalomyelitis relates to the possible effect on the brain and spinal cord. This term may suggest that there is inflammation of the central nervous tissue. However, with ME/CFS, inflammation of the spinal cord is not always present.

Chapter 2

Defining ME/CFS

Chronic fatigue syndrome (CFS) or myalgic encephalomyelitis (ME), as it has been known in the UK since an outbreak in 1955 at London's Royal Free Hospital, was first identified by consultant physician in infectious diseases, Dr Melvyn Ramsay. It is a clinically accepted condition now referred to in the UK as ME/CFS. As the suffix '-itis' means inflammation of some kind, some health professionals now use the term 'myalgic encephalomyelopathy', signifying a disease state within the head and the spine but not necessarily accompanied by inflammation.

The name chronic fatigue syndrome is used by most medical practitioners around the world, although most patients I meet prefer the term ME (myalgic encephalomyelitis/ myalgic encephalomyelopathy) as this implies a disease state and is much more than just fatigue. However, the term ME by itself is not widely used except in the UK, Norway and Canada and can lead to confusion and may substantially undermine the progress that has been made by many scientists' original research into CFS.

The joint term ME/CFS was agreed upon by the UK's independent working group in its report to the Chief Medical Officer, Sir Liam Donaldson, published on 11 January 2002 into the condition, so I have used it in my work, but there is still much debate over the most suitable name. Patient groups in the UK prefer the term ME, whereas on my travels I have learnt that some countries have never heard of ME, but they do know of CFS.

In 2007, Canadian physician Dr Bruce M Carruthers and colleagues published a new working case definition of ME/CFS. It was the first set of criteria for the diagnosis of ME/CFS rather than the less specific CFS. This clinical case definition has been updated to what is now known as the International Consensus Criteria (ICC), which is gradually being accepted around the world, and states that, in order to be diagnosed with ME/CFS, the patient:

- must become symptomatically ill after physical or mental exertion.

- must have signs and symptoms, other than fatigue, such as neurological, neurocognitive, neuroendocrine and/or immune manifestations and signs of autonomic disturbance.

Fibromyalgia

Fibromyalgia, also known as fibromyalgia syndrome (FMS), was first observed by Dr William Balfour in 1824, who described 'tender points', which were then examined in detail by French physician François Valliex in 1841. It was referred to as 'fibrositis' in the *British Medical Journal* in 1904 by British neurologist, Sir William Garvey. However, the term wrongly implied that the pain and discomfort were due to inflammation. The more correct term fibromyalgia has been used since 1976.

Fibromyalgia is viewed by many as a form of ME/CFS, but with severe widespread pain in all four quadrants of the body (see Figure 7 opposite) being the principal symptom.

From 1990 until 2010, the American College of Rheumatology (ACR) classified fibromyalgia based on the existence of 11 of 18 tender points on the body known as the fibromyalgia trigger points. However, the problem with these tender points was that some doctors pressed too hard and virtually all patients were diagnosed as having fibromyalgia, while some doctors pressed too little, with hardly any diagnoses consequently being made. Also, many patients were being pressed in the wrong places, and so in 2010 the ACR developed new criteria for the diagnosis of fibromyalgia.

According to the present information from the ACR, fibromyalgia is a neurologic chronic health condition that causes pain in all four quadrants of the body if one divided the body into segments, plus many other symptoms similar to ME/CFS.

The criteria do not account for people having another disorder at the same time (known as comorbidity) which unfortunately can happen and does so quite often, especially with ME/CFS, which also leads to general muscle pain (myalgia). The

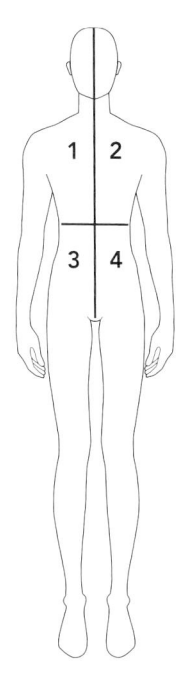

Fig. 7 The main feature of fibromyalgia is pain in all four quadrants of the body.

symptoms of FMS are very similar to those of ME/CFS and this is why I feel they are on the same spectrum of the disease process, with FMS being diagnosed when there is widespread severe pain in all parts of the body, not just aching muscles or minor discomfort. For years, FMS was considered a rheumatologic disorder; however, the immune system has been shown to be important in the pathological process of this disease. There is much evidence to show that FMS, like ME/CFS, also arises from disturbed connections between the central autonomic nervous system, the hormonal system and the immune system.

Conclusion

ME/CFS and FMS are two very similar conditions that are due to a disturbance of the lymphatic drainage of the central nervous system. This leads to a disturbed sympathetic nervous system which causes further imbalance of overall body functions leading to the many symptoms seen in these disorders. Since there are no proven blood or other lab tests for ME/CFS and FMS, they are generally diagnosed after all other possible conditions have been excluded.

Chapter 3

The role of toxins in ME/CFS and FMS

The word 'toxin' was coined in the late nineteenth century and is defined as 'an antigenic poison or venom of plant or animal origin, especially one produced or derived from micro-organisms and causing disease when present at low concentrations in the body'. For simplicity, 'toxin' is used in this book in the broader sense of any substance that is harmful to the body. Accordingly, mercury, which is a heavy-metal toxin, is from neither plant nor animal source but is nevertheless a major toxin to the body. Nowadays there are many man-made toxins, including chemical weapons such as novichok, which is Russian for 'newcomer' but has been around since the 1970s. We definitely have a lot more to contend with today than in the 1800s!

Pollutants

Environmental pollutants have long been seen as major causative factors in neurodegenerative disorders, such as Parkinson's disease, although there may also be genetic factors that make a person more susceptible to that illness. Studies have revealed major variations in an individual's ability to detoxify noxious agents and have shown that neurological disease may derive from an exceptional vulnerability to certain neurotoxins.

Amazingly, with over 144,000 chemicals in the environment, less than two dozen have actually been banned. The US Government Office of Technology has estimated that up to 25% of all chemicals might be neurotoxic. The US Department of Health has estimated that each year approximately 2000 new chemicals are produced and, no matter what safety procedures are taken, they are all – inadvertently or deliberately – introduced into the environment via the air, water or foodstuffs.

According to Julian Cribb, author of *Surviving the 21st Century*, more than 250 billion tonnes of chemical substances a year are harming people and life everywhere on the planet. Worse still, according to the World Health Organization, around 12 million people die every year from diseases caused by the direct and indirect impact of man-made pollutants.

The figures per year are frightening:

- 30 million tonnes of manufactured chemicals produced per year
- 400 million tonnes of hazardous waste are generated per year
- Over 11 billion tonnes of coal, oil and gas are burned per year.

Not to mention the hundreds of billions of tonnes of waste products that are found in water and the food chain worldwide. Environmental pollutants have been discovered at the top of Mount Everest and at the bottom of the deepest oceans. Mercury is seen in the tissue of polar bears in the Arctic, and honeybees are dying globally from agricultural pesticides.

The sources of toxic exposure, such as benzene from motor fuels, organophosphates in pesticides, chlorofluorocarbons (CFCs) in cleaning products and carbon monoxide, have been implicated as potential causative factors of ME/CFS. However, as one can see from the above figures, these are just the tip of the toxic iceberg that globally pervades our environment.

Effects of neurotoxins

Toxic chemical exposure can cause many serious conditions, including cardiovascular, kidney and endocrine diseases. The most common organ to be affected by toxins, however, is the brain, leading to fatigue, exhaustion, cognitive impairment, loss of memory, insomnia, depression, psychosis and other disturbing symptoms.

As mentioned earlier, there are several specialised regions in the brain that do not have a complete blood–brain barrier (BBB) and which interact closely with the cerebrospinal fluid. These zones are chemical-sensitive regions that may react with toxins, sending messages to other parts of the brain, especially the hypothalamus.

The hypothalamus controls the hormonal (endocrine) system via a mechanism called biofeedback. Basically, the hypothalamus 'tastes' the blood to check how much hormone needs to be released into the circulation. It then sends messages to endocrine organs around the body to increase or decrease levels of the many different hormones. Since hormones are made up of large protein molecules, the BBB, which normally protects against large toxic molecules, is extremely permeable in the region of the hypothalamus. This allows the passage of specific protein-transport molecules that enable huge molecules to pass through the BBB. Thus, the most permeable region of the BBB is at the hypothalamus, facilitating its ability to monitor hormone levels in the blood.

Autonomic dysfunction has long been associated with many toxic substances, especially following exposure to organic solvents, with some people exhibiting signs and symptoms of peripheral neuropathy (nerve damage in the limbs, hands and feet).

Under normal conditions, most of the BBB protects the central nervous system from rapid fluctuations in levels of ions, neurotransmitters, bacterial toxins, growth factors and other substances. However, its permeability has been shown to be increased by stress.

Each organ or tissue may act as a discrete target for some toxic substances, which may lead to dysfunction of the whole organism. Specific molecules within a particular cell type act as primary targets. Some neurons are less susceptible than others to toxic damage, leading to regions of the brain that are not as sensitive to toxins.

Diet and toxicity

Exposure to chemicals affects people in different ways depending on several factors. Diet plays a crucial part in the body's ability to withstand toxicity. Toxins can be produced from non-toxic foods that we eat, building up in the central nervous system, liver or kidneys.

Trace elements, which are often used as supplements for good health, may become toxic if ingested in too high a dose. One thinks of selenium, for example, as a promoter of health, but it may be taken up from the soil by certain plants, such as species of the *Astralagus* genus, in sufficient quantities to render those plants toxic. Chronic selenium poisoning in animals, known as alkali disease, leads to cases of livestock with lameness, lack of vitality, hair loss, depressed appetite and emaciation.

Healthy food may not be properly digested or absorbed. The person may have a leaky gut due to problems with the intestinal wall, leading to semi-digested food entering the bloodstream, causing immune responses which create further toxicity. Even fruit and vegetables, especially non-organic ones bought in supermarkets around the world, often contain a cocktail of toxic chemical preservatives and enhancements which will aggravate the situation.

Damage to the lining of the alimentary canal (gut) may be caused by a variety of irritants, the most common being alcohol, aspirin, gluten and the yeast *Candida albicans*. Deficiencies in some vitamins, proteins, essential fatty acids and minerals are known to lead to poor intestinal cell growth, causing increased permeability of the gut wall. The gut's microbiome (resident bacteria and other microbes) is essential for the production of most of the chemicals used by the nervous system.

Toxins in the gut can destroy many of the 'good' bacteria and render the body incapable of producing the essential neuropeptides necessary for a healthy brain. This further exacerbates the toxic soup building up in the central nervous system in ME/CFS and FMS.

Predisposition to toxicity

Previous exposure to toxins will increase an individual's sensitivity to further toxic insult (attack). Some people have a greater genetic ability to detoxify while, unfortunately, others are more likely to experience more severe symptoms from toxic causes due to their individual genetic predisposition. Likewise, one's prior state of health, with the emphasis on the immune system, is a major significant factor to consider when assessing human ability to withstand exposure to poisonous chemicals. Age is important, with children much more susceptible to toxic overload than adults, because of their faster rate of absorption and smaller body weight – hence the smaller dosages of prescribed medicines allowed to children.

Several chemicals have the potential to induce autoimmune diseases such as systemic lupus erythematosus, commonly known as 'lupus' or 'SLE'.

Genetic susceptibilities have been discovered in diseases such as autoimmune hepatitis. The immune profile and genetic predisposition in some ME/CFS sufferers is likely to render these individuals more prone to toxic attack. This has been termed 'ecogenetics'.

Also, let us not forget epigenetics, where gene expression can change due to external influences, such as increased toxins. Important genetic research is taking place in the USA on people with neuroimmune disorders and looking at a possible genetic predisposition to ME/CFS. With the largest ever genetic study on 20,000 ME/CFS patients, which began in the UK in 2020, scientists hope to learn much more about genetic predisposition to this disease.

Conclusion

Our bodies are constantly under siege by thousands of poisonous agents, yet many of us remain healthy. The reason for this is that the healthy body is able to drain the toxins away from the brain. If this drainage system is not working properly and/or pumping the fluid in the wrong direction, problems will arise, and if the neuro-lymphatic system is dysfunctional, neuro-immune illnesses such as ME/CFS, fibromyalgia, and most probably Lyme disease, Gulf War syndrome and Alzheimer's, plus many other unexplained illnesses affecting the central nervous system, will occur.

Chapter 4

The stages leading to ME/CFS and FMS

With careful consideration of over 30 years of clinical and research findings, I have established a theoretical model to explain the cause, signs and symptoms of ME/CFS and the effectiveness of my treatment regime. My belief is that my approach does not set out directly to eliminate poisons from the body; rather, it facilitates the patient's own in-built mechanisms responsible for toxin elimination.

First a few facts that you need to know about the nervous system.

The nervous system can be divided into the central and peripheral systems. The central nervous system consists of the brain and the spinal cord, the peripheral system, which spreads out to the rest of the body, is further subdivided into the somatic and the autonomic nervous systems.

The somatic nervous system is associated with the voluntary control of body movements via motor nerves controlling the skeletal muscles plus sensory nerves receiving information from all over the body. The autonomic nervous system, on the other hand, regulates a variety of body processes that take place without conscious effort, as described in Chapter 2.

The autonomic nervous system is further divided into separate systems. The main one related to ME/CFS and FMS is the sympathetic nervous system, which makes the body ready for the 'fight or flight' response during any impending threat as described on page 11. On the other hand, the parasympathetic nervous system inhibits the body from overworking and restores it to a calm and composed state but can be also involved in the disease process as explained in more detail in Chapter 3 (page 73) in *The Perrin Technique 2nd Edition*.

By reducing the intensity of incoming sympathetic activity, by means of relaxing the muscles and improving circulation and drainage, the signs and symptoms of ME/CFS and FMS gradually diminish. My theoretical model of the stages of development of ME/CFS (see Table 4.1) reflects the clinical history of all the ME/CFS and FMS patients I have seen since the late 1980s.

Table 4.1 The stages of development leading to ME/CFS and FMS

Stage 1	Patients with ME/CFS and FMS all seem to have a predisposing history of sympathetic nervous system overload:
a	Physically – by being an overachiever at work, during study, or in sports. Rarely, it may be the opposite by being too sedentary.
b	Chemically – by constant exposure to environmental pollution.
c	Immunologically – by chronic infections or hypersensitivities to multiple allergens.
d	Psychologically/emotionally – by family and/or work-related mental stress.
Stage 2	In Stage 2 either a or b can occur before the other or they can occur concurrently, depending on the causes of the restricted flow of lymphatic drainage in the head and spine.
a	Lymphatic drainage from the brain shows signs of being impaired, mostly in the cribriform plate region of the ethmoid bone above the nasal passages, the neural pathways along the optic nerve behind the eye, the trigeminal pathways in the region of the upper jaw and the drainage along auditory pathways.
b	Lymphatic drainage of the central nervous system is also subject to disturbances in the spine, usually in the cervical or thoracic region, due to either a congenital, hereditary or postural defect and/or prior trauma.

Stage 3	Toxic effects due to the long-term dysfunction of the central nervous system drainage will compound the chronic hyperactivity of the sympathetic nervous system; this further overloads the hypothalamus and subsequently, the sympathetic nervous system.
Stage 4	A final trigger factor strikes, which usually arises from a viral infection, but may be physical, chemical or emotional in nature.
Stage 5	There will be a disturbance in autonomic, as well as hormonal, function, because toxins in the cerebral blood flow and ventricular system directly affect control of the hypothalamus. Hormonal transport within the cerebrospinal fluid may be directly affected by toxic overload.
Stage 6	Dysfunction of sympathetic control of the lymphatics, especially the thoracic duct, leads to a reflux of toxins in the resultant retrograde lymph flow, causing varicose lymphatic vessels (see Figure 13) predominantly in the neck, chest and abdomen. This also further reduces flow of cerebrospinal fluid into the lymphatics.
Stage 7	Further backflow of toxic drainage into the central nervous system, due to the retrograde lymphatics, results in increased hypothalamic dysfunction and an even greater disturbance of lymphatic drainage.
Stage 8	The continuing irritation of the sympathetic nervous system results in further systemic disturbances, leading to chronic adaptive states known as ME/CFS and FMS.

The physical signs of ME/CFS and FMS

I once had the pleasure of hearing a Stanford Professor of Medicine, Dr Abraham Verghese, at an international ME/CFS conference in California who made the most profound statement: 'The Doctor's round ... has become square'. In other words, instead of physically examining the patient, as in days gone by, most physicians are busy looking at a screen for pathological tests etc; in most cases, they should also be looking at and listening to the patient to work out what is really going on. As a trained osteopath, I listen to, observe and palpate all patients before making any diagnosis. Sometimes pathological tests and computers are needed to confirm the diagnosis, but one should always carry out a physical examination first. As I have said, many patients who suffer from ME/CFS are left untreated, with the physician hoping that the patient will spontaneously recover, learn to live with the problem, or change doctors. Despite the fact that the World Health Organization (WHO) has recognised myalgic encephalomyelitis (ME) as a neurological disease since at least 1969, and despite thousands of scientific papers being published which demonstrate that ME/CFS is a real physical disease, with many different pathological findings, there are still many GPs who refuse to believe in a physical source of the symptoms and refer their patients to a psychiatrist.

Although many in the medical profession now recognise the category ME/CFS and realise that there is something physically wrong with the patient, they do not know how to diagnose or how to treat it. Most of my patients who suffer from this condition have been to neurologists, undergone brain scans, X-rays, blood tests and many other exhaustive examinations, all of which have yielded inconclusive evidence that there is anything wrong at all. This may lead to the patient being told to get on with life as best they can and to try and forget about their symptoms. The usual advice given to sufferers is to rest until the body sorts itself out, or worse, to increase activity, which mostly causes the patient's symptoms to quickly deteriorate. Sadly, in many cases patients end up forgotten by their healthcare providers as they spend months and often years bed-ridden in darkened rooms, in silence with little communication with the outside world; this can hardly be called 'living'. Many ME/CFS and fibromyalgia patients just exist, waiting for the miracle cure that never comes. Even more depressing is that often the patients' own family and friends do not give the patient the support they need. Even in cases where the patient does have a loving and caring family and group of friends, there is a lack of understanding regarding both ME/CFS and fibromyalgia. This lack of understanding is compounded by the media, which often belittles these diseases as just 'in the mind' and suggests that these patients are actually not that ill. How many 'get well' cards are ever received by ME/CFS or fibromyalgia patients? … Usually none!

The concept of ME/CFS being primarily a biophysical rather than a psychological disorder is foreign to most of the medical profession. However, many doctors recognise that ME/CFS causes physical signs and symptoms. Physical components have always been included in the internationally recognised criteria that verify the diagnosis of ME/CFS. These include sore throat, tender lymph nodes in the neck and armpits, and muscle and joint pain.

In the 32 years since I started to examine and treat patients with ME/CFS, and indeed FMS, repeated patterns of physical signs have emerged among all the sufferers that cannot be dismissed as pure coincidence. All physical phenomena seen in ME/CFS can be understood when the disease is viewed as the consequence of impaired drainage of the central nervous system coupled with a dysfunction of the sympathetic nervous system. This is explained in detail in the large, expanded *The Perrin Technique 2nd Edition*.

These signs have been confirmed in a recent NHS study at Wrightington Hospital and were published in the online version of *The British Medical Journal* in November 2017 (see Chapter 8, page 253 in the *2nd Edition*). These signs have also been present in the FMS patients I have seen over my many years in practice, which is another reason I feel the two conditions share a common pathophysiology, the main difference being that FMS patients compared with ME/CFS patients have more intense and widespread pain in all parts of the body. The main physical signs are shown in Figure 8.

The following five regions of tenderness or dysfunction have been identified in virtually all ME/CFS sufferers that I have seen since 1989 in both the university and clinical settings.

1. Longstanding thoracic (upper back) spinal problems
2. Varicose lymphatics
3. Tenderness in the left breast at a point now referred to as Perrin's Point
4. Tenderness in an area at the upper mid-section of the abdomen known as the coeliac or solar plexus
5. Disturbance in the cranial rhythmic impulse (cranial-sacral rhythm).

The Perrin Technique

1. Longstanding thoracic spinal problems (often with flatness, redness, heat or pain in the mid-thoracic spine)
2. Varicose lymphatics
3. Perrin's Point
4. Coeliac plexus (solar plexus) tenderness
5. Abnormal cranio-sacral rhythm (cranial rhythmic impulse)

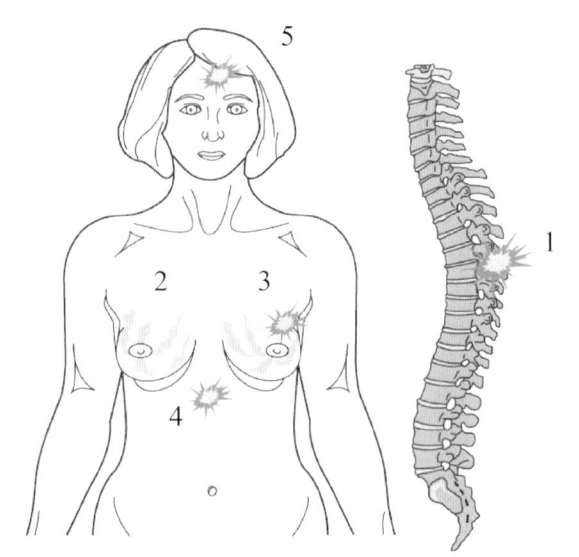

Fig. 8 The observed physical signs of ME/CFS.

1. Longstanding thoracic (upper back) spinal problems

A prevailing observation in the clinical findings of ME/CFS is a mechanical disorder of the thoracic spine, which may be due to bad occupational posture, or related to a congenital event or genetic predisposition or injury.

There is much truth in the famous song *Dry Bones* by the Delta Rhythm Boys, you know the one which has the immortal lines:

'Your toe bone connected to your foot bone
'Your foot bone connected to your heel bone ...'

and so on and so on until we get to the top of the body …

'Your back bone connected to your shoulder bone
'Your shoulder bone connected to your neck bone
'Your neck bone connected to your head bone
'I hear the word of the Lord.'

Chapter 4

What this reminds us of is that any physical (genetic or otherwise) defect in one part of the body can have a major influence on another section. For instance, if one has one leg slightly shorter than the other it will lead to a compensatory lateral shift in the spinal column causing possible drainage problems in the spinal perivascular pathways and extra strain on the surrounding soft tissue, which includes the muscles, ligaments and fascia. This can then create extra pressure on the blood and lymph vessel walls, causing disturbed circulation and drainage. Likewise, an upper spinal problem can create a disparity in the forces placed on the legs and feet. This actually happened in clinic when a girl came in wearing callipers on her left lower leg. This was due to a weakness in her left ankle that for years had baffled her doctors. I discovered an upper spinal scoliosis (side-bending) that placed too much pressure on her left side, leading to eventual pain in the left leg, foot and ankle. Over the years she had compensated for the pain by using her right dominant side much more, resulting in the eventual weakness in her left ankle and foot requiring support.

Another case that illustrates the genetic predisposition to postural related problems was a boy with ME/CFS who was tongue-tied at birth which was a familial complaint. The tethered oral tissue when born tongue-tied can lead to the head being tilted low and forward. This stooped posture can affect the neuro-lymphatic drainage of the spine and surrounding soft tissue with the resultant neurological and circulatory dysfunction.

The most common structural disturbance that I have seen in ME/CFS and FMS patients is a flattening of the curvature in the mid-thoracic spine, usually accompanied by the presence of a kyphotic dorso-lumbar area (an abnormally exaggerated convex curvature in the lower back). An example of this defect is shown in Figure 9a which can be compared with the healthy posture shown in Figure 9b. This postural defect is often caused by a prior condition, spinal osteochondrosis, also known as Scheuermann's disease, which affects spinal development in adolescence, and which may have occurred years before the onset of the characteristic symptoms of ME/CFS and FMS.

Also, when one feels the skin lying over the thoracic spine, it is usually hotter (but not always) than other regions of the trunk, which may indicate an underlying area

The Perrin Technique

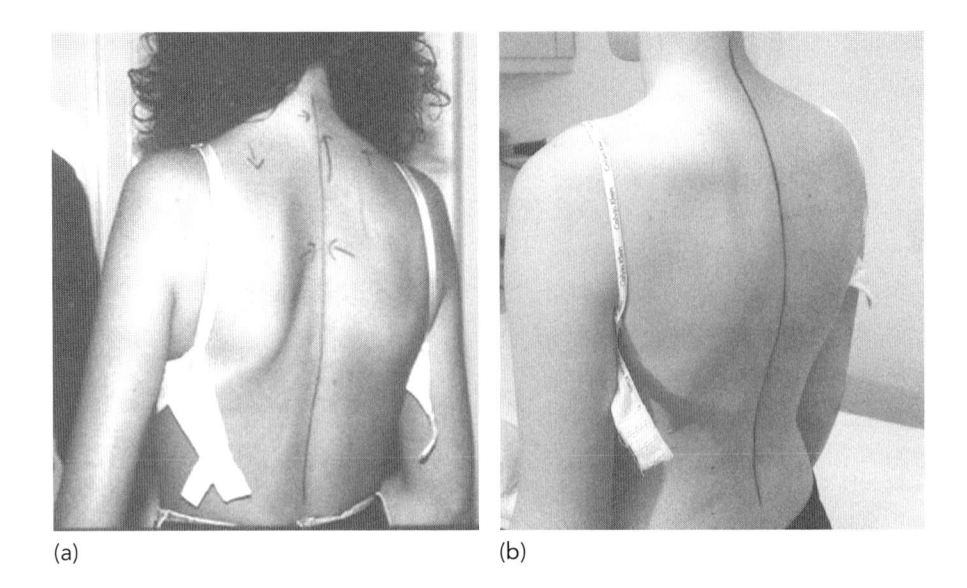

Fig. 9 Comparative photographs showing a flattened mid-thoracic spine. Photo (a) shows the familiar flattening of the mid-thoracic spine seen in many ME/CFS and FMS patients. This differs from a normal spinal posture in the healthy subject, photo (b).

of inflammation. Another common finding in this region in ME/CFS and FMS is the presence of trophic changes – that is, changes due to interruption of the nerve supply which affects nerve interactions with other cells, such as the skin, leading to molecular changes, including dryness, spots and rashes. Scars are also sometimes seen, indicating previous injury or surgery in the region. Also, abnormal amounts of redness in the skin overlying this region of the back is often seen after it is stimulated by a rubbing/stroking motion. (There is a colour photograph of this in *The Perrin Technique 2nd Edition*.)

2. Varicose lymphatics and 3. Perrin's Point

In every ME/CFS patient, whether male or female, there is a tender area in the upper lateral region of the breast tissue, roughly 2 cm superior and lateral to the left nipple (see Figures 8 (marked with a '3') and 10). This finding is significant because the tender area almost always lies on the left side and is level with the position at which the thoracic duct turns to the left. The heart and the main blood vessels are supplied with sympathetic nerves via a bundle of nerves called the cardiac plexus, which has a greater concentration of nerves on the left than the right. Sympathetic nerves that are close to the skin run alongside the larger nerves that control movement and sensation in the body (the somatic nerves). Impulses cross over from sympathetic nerves to somatic sensory nerves and vice versa between the adjacent parallel nerve fibres via what are called ephapses.

When the cardiac rhythm is affected in ME/CFS, the sympathetic nerves send messages to the sensory nerves on the left side of the chest. The thoracic duct travels from the right side to the left side of body above the level of the nipple and so sympathetic nerves controlling the thoracic duct's pumping action are more left-sided above the nipple line. Thus, when these nerves are irritated, they also disturb the adjacent sensory nerves. The resultant pain is at the confluence of these two networks of irritated sensory nerves. This tender spot is now known as 'Perrin's Point' (see the 'X' in Figure 10). In FMS this point is usually extremely tender, much more so than in the standard ME/CFS patient.

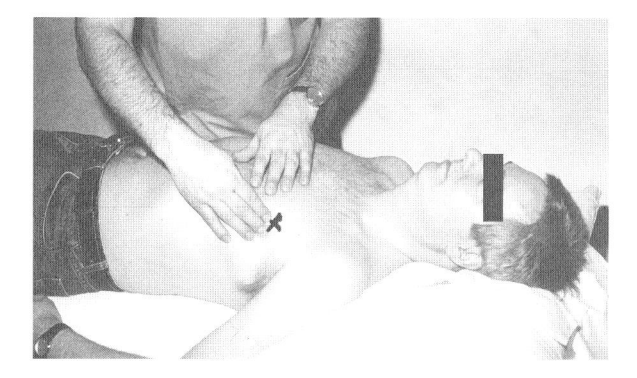

Fig. 10 Examining a male patient for 'Perrin's Point'. Gentle pressure at a point slightly superior and lateral to the left nipple, 'Perrin's Point'(**X**). The amount of sensitivity at this point appears to correspond to the severity of lymphatic engorgement in the breast tissue and also seems to mirror the gravity of the other symptoms.

Since the 1990s I have felt the sensitive region now known as Perrin's Point, together with congested lymph vessels in the cervical (neck) region and breast tissue, in nearly all the thousands of ME/CFS patients I have examined. The consistency of these lymphatics can best be described as a 'string of beads' and similar to varicose veins in the leg. Varicosities have been described before in the lymphatic system. Large incompetent varicose lymphatics, known as 'megalymphatics', have often been seen when there is a backflow of fluid within the lymphatic vessels, due to a disturbance of the normal pumping mechanism. However, varicosities in the lymphatics are rarely discussed in clinics, due to the misconception that lymph flow can only be unidirectional due to a system of valves in the lymphatic vessels. Sluggish lymph flow is known to exist in many disease states and is treated by many practitioners worldwide, trained in manual lymphatic drainage. However, the concept of a reverse pump causing an actual backflow is not generally recognised clinically. Thus, the possibility of a varicose lymph vessel is rarely considered when a GP or hospital consultant conducts an examination.

Downward pressure due to thoracic duct pump dysfunction caused by sympathetic disequilibrium may lead to a contra-flow within the lymphatics, damaging the valves and creating a pooling of lymphatic fluid with exaggerated 'beading' of the vessels. Stasis (fluid not moving) in these varicose lymphatic vessels creates a risk of toxic overload together with additional damage to the lymphatics and surrounding tissue.

Reflux of toxins via lymphatic vessels back into the cerebrospinal fluid will further irritate the central nervous system. Increased toxicity within the central nervous system continues to overload the sympathetic nerves, resulting in a downward spiral of deteriorating health.

From the earliest days of osteopathy, the importance of good lymphatic drainage in the thoracic duct has been seen as paramount to sustain health. It was emphasised that, together with good blood supply, it was equally important to have perfect drainage. This is the pathway I believe to be compromised mechanically as part of the root cause of ME/CFS. Mechanical dysfunction such as this can be detected by palpation with the finger tips and can be released by gentle pressure and massage techniques applied to the cranium and the spine and surrounding soft tissue.

The healthy lymphatic vessel allows only unidirectional flow due to the system of valves illustrated in Figure 11.

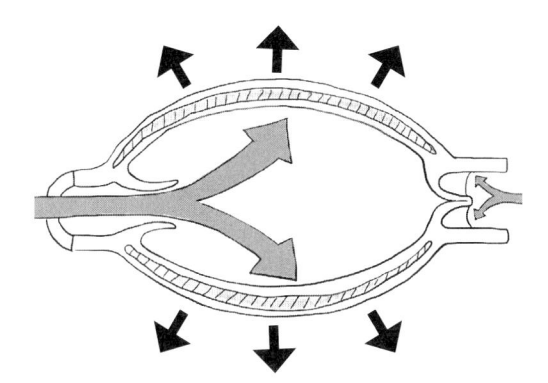

Fig. 11 Schematic illustration showing normal flow within a healthy lymphatic vessel. The valves in this healthy vessel are intact, preventing any backflow, thus maintaining a healthy, unidirectional drainage (note the smooth muscular wall of the lymphangion regulated by sympathetic nerves).

In ME/CFS and FMS, retrograde flow of the lymphatics is produced by the reverse peristaltic wave of the thoracic duct that arises from dysfunctional sympathetic control of the duct's smooth muscle wall. This causes a reflux of fluid throughout the lymphatic system affecting individual lymph-collecting vessels (lymphangia), leading to the formation of varicose megalymphatics, initially in the neck and chest, as seen in Figure 12a–c. Eventually, the lymphatic reflux causes damage to the valves and allows pooling of fluid in between them (Figure 12b). This leads to distension of the vessel wall with the characteristic enlarged beaded appearance of a varicose vessel as illustrated in Figure 12c.

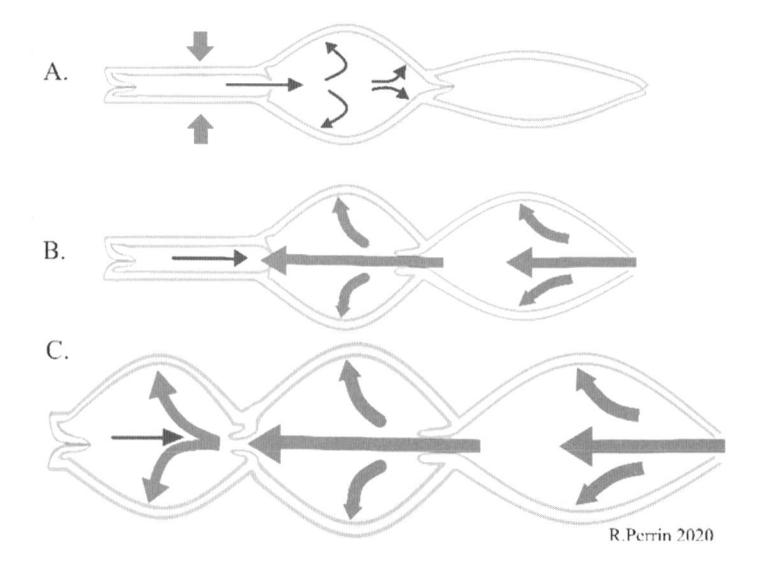

Fig. 12 The development of varicose megalymphatics (a) The normal lymph flow before the illness. (b) Reversal of the central lymphatic pump forces the colourless lymph fluid back, damaging the valves that separate the adjacent collecting vessels (lymphangia). (c) The lymphangia expand due to the pressure and volume of the backward flowing lymph. This leads to the large beaded vessels (varicose mega-lymphatics) palpated (felt with the fingertips) just beneath the skin in the chest of ME/CFS and FMS patients.

Figure 13 shows the top right section of the chest of a 61-year-old man. One can see the swollen, tortuous beaded vessels just beneath the collar bone adjacent to the right shoulder. The man suffered severely from ME/CFS for four years before being successfully treated with a two-year course of the Perrin Technique. The beaded appearance in Figure 13 is due to damaged valves and subsequent retrograde flow and pooling of lymphatic fluid. This is similar to the formation of varicose veins, although it lacks the darker, bluish hue of superficial varicose veins. The fluid in the lymphatic vessel, known simply as 'lymph', is colourless and so these vessels are definitely lymphatic and not blood vessels as they have the same colour as the overlying skin. (A colour version of this photograph appears in *The Perrin Technique 2nd Edition*.) These vessels also have a much larger diameter than do healthy superficial lymphatic vessels, which are normally extremely difficult to palpate, never mind actually see with the naked eye. It is extremely rare to see such pronounced superficial varicose megalymphatics as illustrated here. However, I have been able to feel the presence of varicose lymphatic vessels in the chests of virtually all the ME/CFS and FMS patients I have seen since 1989.

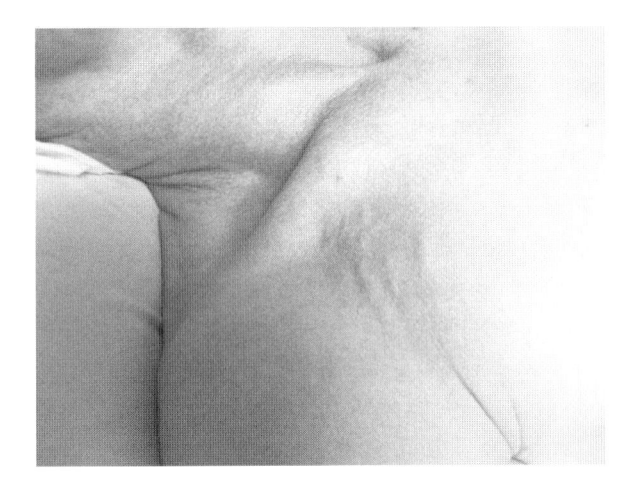

Fig. 13 Right subclavicular varicose megalymphatics, lacking the bluish hue of varicose veins, in a patient with ME/CFS.

4. Tenderness at the coeliac or solar plexus

The largest major plexus of the autonomic nervous system, uniting two large coeliac ganglia, is known as the **coeliac plexus**, more commonly referred to as the 'solar plexus' (see Figure 8).

Through its connections, the solar plexus is excellent as an indicator for any visceral disturbances from the waist down. Tenderness in this abdominal region, known as the epigastrium, seems to be directly related to the severity of any lower extremity fatigue and/or abdominal problem. This, as with Perrin's Point, is due to impulses passing across the 'ephapses' – connections between adjacent sensory and sympathetic nerves – and, again, is usually much more tender in FMS patients.

On palpation, the epigastrium is also usually warmer than the rest of the abdomen, possibly due to the back flow of inflammatory toxins pumping down the thoracic duct into the upper regions of the abdomen and also the build-up of neurogenic inflammation from coeliac plexus overload.

5. Disturbance in the cranio-sacral rhythm

There is a palpable rhythmic pulsation along the spinal cord and around the brain together with that of normal breathing, which is transmitted to the rest of the body and is termed the cranial rhythmic impulse (CRI) or the 'cranio-sacral rhythm'. The rhythm is also known by some osteopaths as the 'involuntary mechanism' and by others as the 'primary respiration' as it is believed by some to be the inherent driver of all other mechanisms and rhythms in the body. Most of the osteopathic profession believe this pulse to be a movement through the tension and continuity of membranes and fascia. The fascia is the name for connective tissue throughout the body containing many lymphatic vessels that is continuous with the membranes that surround the brain and spinal cord, the meninges, thus allowing the different motions, and tensions, of the body to be transmitted everywhere.

William Garner Sutherland (1873–1954), the founder of cranial osteopathy, proposed that there was a primary respiratory mechanism created within the central nervous system and via the spinal cord, with the bones in the cranium all moving in a rhythmic pattern together with the sacrum at the base of the spine.

Sutherland proposed that the primary respiratory mechanism produces a rhythmic alternation of flexion and extension of structures in the midline. This movement occurs simultaneously with rhythmic external and internal rotation of all paired lateral structures.

Lymphatic vessels with muscular walls that expand and contract exist throughout the body, which creates a powerful pumping mechanism. It has been shown that the thoracic duct pump influences the drainage of CSF/lymph from the central nervous system. Together with the pulse rate and the effects of breathing, a separate underlying rhythm may be induced which is very possibly the aforementioned 'involuntary mechanism'. This rhythm echoes along the lymphatic system, resonating throughout the entire body and can be palpated (felt) by trained practitioners. In ME/CFS and FMS patients it is often slower, arrhythmic, plus its intensity is shallower than in healthy people, and in very severe cases it is almost absent. A disturbed CRI was found in all the ME/CFS patients that I have examined clinically and during my research.

My theory is that the CRI is produced by the drainage of cerebrospinal fluid from the brain and spine into the lymphatics. It is a product of the two dynamic fluid systems, each with its own distinct rhythm, coming together to produce this third cranial rhythm, similar to a large incoming wave on a beach colliding with a much shallower wave going out, creating a third wave.

My theory is also supported by the fact that CSF drainage into the lymphatics in humans has now been proven and that neuroscientists have shown that breathing and posture affect the movement of CSF and thus aid CSF drainage to the lymphatics.

The two minor physical signs

Over the years I have observed two other notable signs that appear in many cases but they are not present in the majority, so I call them the minor physical signs. These are stretch marks and pupil dilation.

- **Stretch marks**, known medically as 'striae', are caused by damaged collagen fibres close to the skin surface. Striae are often seen on the thighs and breast tissue of ME/CFS patients and are most probably due to damage to collagenous anchoring ligaments attached to surface lymphatic vessels. This could occur when there is a major backflow of lymph and is seen in many ME/CFS patients who have never been obese or pregnant, which are the two most common physiological causes of striae.

- **Pupil dilation.** In ME/CFS and FMS, due to dysfunction of the sympathetic nervous system, the size of the patient's pupils can be grossly affected. Some patients have reduced sympathetic nerve activity leading to pupil constriction but having dilated pupils due to sympathetic overload is much more frequent, with the patient needing to avoid bright lights and sunshine. Some ME/CFS and FMS patients need to wear sunglasses all the time, with the worst cases so photophobic that they need to wear blackout eye masks.

Scoring the patient

After scrutinising your symptoms and medical history and following the physical examination a practitioner trained in the Perrin Technique should be able to calculate if you indeed have ME/CFS and/or FMS and also be able to give an initial score out of 10, with 10/10 being symptom-free (see the outlook chart, Table 5.3, Chapter 5, page 89). Taking into account the number of different symptoms, the practitioner will be able to provide a definitive score once the physical examination has been carried out. This will confirm whether a person is exaggerating their symptoms, which I must add is very rare with ME/CFS and FMS, or if they are playing down their symptoms and acting as though they are healthier than the five signs indicate. This is much more common with ME/CFS and FMS patients, who hate the fact that they are suffering from such a debilitating illness which most people, including their healthcare practitioners, don't understand.

So, ME/CFS sufferers often pretend to all their family and friends that they can do much more than they can actually manage, at a terrible cost to themselves as it inevitably leads to a steady deterioration of the symptoms. Many patients who I see for the initial consultation fall into this category and there is a massive group of the 'three-and-a-half out of 10' patients acting like a 'seven out of 10'. They are often wives and mothers who need to, or have to, carry on to try and keep the home as normal as possible for their spouses and children, as they feel desperately guilty if they admit how bad their illness is, or try and rest more and pace themselves better. ME/CFS isn't the worst illness there is, but it is one of the cruellest. It usually affects people with very strong willpower who are extremely active before and will try and beat the disease with every fibre in their body and with *über* determination. However, the more they try and beat the disease, the worse they get. The sympathetic nervous system is the main control mechanism of the neuro-immune system and it is this connection that needs to function properly to enable willpower to beat disease.

There are plenty of practitioners trained in cranio-sacral techniques who can apply all the above diagnostic procedures that may identify ME/CFS in its earliest stages.

In fact, clinically when examining siblings or children of ME/CFS patients, I have discovered that the physical signs often appear long before the symptoms present themselves fully. This being the case in patients with a familial predisposition, it is possible in these instances to actually diagnose a pre-ME/CFS condition and prevent certain patients from ever succumbing to the full-blown illness. As far as I know, I am the only clinician to claim that ME/CFS is preventable.

In May/June 2020 I treated a 42-year-old man from Prestwich, Manchester, who until recently had had no previous history of ME/CFS symptoms. However, since he had been infected by Covid-19 in the spring of 2020, he had felt overwhelming physical and mental fatigue with many other symptoms of ME/CFS. He lived near my clinic and knew of my work so made an appointment to see me. On examination, his physical signs were prominent and clearly palpable, with mid-thoracic tenderness, huge varicose lymphatics, very tender Perrin's Point and coeliac plexus plus very 'sluggish' CRI. After only three treatments the physical signs began to fade, and his symptoms improved. A couple of months on and he was completely symptom-free and back to full health.

The sooner that a patient receives a physical examination with confirmation of the definitive signs and symptoms of neuro-lymphatic dysfunction, the better. This hopefully will lead to a much quicker initiation of treatment than normal. The earlier the treatment programme begins, the better the chances of recovery and the less likely it is that the patient will start to spiral into the chronic severe state that blights so many ME/CFS and FMS sufferers' lives.

Conclusion

This chapter has shown that ME/CFS and FMS are both caused by a dysfunction of the healthy flow of the neuro-lymphatic system due to disturbed spinal mechanics and cranial structure. This in turn leads to the toxic overload of the central nervous system. The vicious circle that ensues eventually leads to these two chronic conditions that can both be diagnosed and treated with the methods shown in this handbook and explained in greater detail in *The Perrin Technique 2nd Edition.*

Chapter 5

Treatment using the Perrin Technique

The magic bullet?

Will there ever be a pill to cure ME/CFS and FMS? This question is raised again and again by patients, doctors and scientists. In my opinion, based on over 30 years of clinical research into this field, unfortunately but unequivocally, NO! This is because every ME/CFS patient and every FMS patient is different, with different toxins affecting different neurochemical pathways, in turn affecting different sections of the central nervous system, causing different metabolic disturbances, leading to a different array of symptoms. This view, as you can imagine, makes me hugely popular at scientific meetings and ME/CFS and FMS conferences … Not!

Of course, nobody wants to hear this, or read this for that matter, and for the patient it looks as if all is lost.

But it isn't!

It just means that we have to approach the treatment of ME/CFS and FMS in a different way to most diseases. As leading Canadian ME/CFS physician, the late Dr Bruce Carruthers, once said, 'Treat the dis-ease and not the disease!'

'Big Pharma', a colloquial term for leading pharmaceutical firms that produce most of our medicines today, don't like to hear this either. If there is not a potential huge return on investment, they may not be motivated in helping research into disease treatment in the first place. If there is little chance of a magic bullet to kill the bug or sort out the biochemical problem, then they won't see the point of funding studies that go on for years and years before any successful pill or potion may be developed. One can hardly blame them – they are commercial organisations.

There are, however, blood and other lab tests and drugs that have been and are being developed that will identify and help some sub-groups of patients, such as targeting an aspect of the immune system or reducing the upregulated stress response. These may help some patients, but unfortunately worsen other individuals with ME/CFS or FMS who have a different symptom picture with other metabolic disturbances.

There are two major and complex problems that continue to beset the diagnosis and treatment of ME/CFS. The first is that two or more conditions can co-exist at any one time in one patient. It is sometimes difficult for doctors to distinguish between, for example, depression and ME/CFS, particularly in those cases of ME/CFS in which depression is an additional feature. The second problem is that, because there is no universally accepted means of diagnosis by tests such as blood or urine analysis, most doctors diagnose ME/CFS by exclusion. In other words, the patient will be diagnosed as suffering from ME/CFS only when all other possible diagnoses have been excluded. In my view, this is a hazardous method of diagnosing any disease. Can you imagine if a doctor were to tell a patient, 'Well, after all the tests, we cannot find anything else wrong with you, so it must be cancer'? Yet thousands of people around the world are being told that they have ME/CFS using the exclusion method of diagnosis.

Some medical experts on ME/CFS have touched upon the neurological effects of the disease, and how the immune system and the body's hormones are affected. However, the treatment recommended by these specialists is to improve the immune system by pharmacological methods or affect the hormonal and chemical balance by dietary means, supplements or hormone replacements and, if necessary, by psychiatric drugs or psychotherapy. These treatments do help symptom relief in many cases and often I will recommend supplementation and agree with many pharmaceutical approaches to help certain symptoms, but if this is all that is done to treat the patient, then these practitioners are missing a crucial point: they are treating just the symptoms rather than aiming at the root cause of the disease. The neurological system that controls the hormonal and chemical balance of the body is the autonomic nervous system and the system that is the main factor in drainage of major toxins from the body as well as a major part of our immune system is the lymphatic system. If these two systems were working correctly, the body would cope with extra stresses and strains due to chemical, physical, mental, immunological and emotional exertion. Only then might pharmacological approaches, psychotherapy and healthy hypoallergenic diets bring about a permanent improvement in patients with ME/CFS.

Sadly, in many people with this condition, there is little or no recovery, despite many and varied dietary and chemical approaches to treatment. The key to finding a complete and lasting remedy is to find a treatment that helps the body cope. This concept is in keeping with modern medicine's approach to the management of other types of disease: for example, the use of vaccinations to increase the body's immunity, and thus resist the effects of certain types of infection.

If one regards any stress factor as an infection, the obvious course of action is to increase the body's defence in staving it off. The fortification of the body is controlled by the autonomic nervous system. The centre of this elaborate web of nerve tissue primarily is found in the hypothalamus and the limbic system of the brain, down to the brain stem, and from the spinal cord spreading throughout the body.

Many sportsmen and women – such as the cyclist Mr E, described at the beginning of Chapter 1 – exert more strain upon their dorsal (thoracic) spine in the pursuit of their sport than the average individual. Golf, yachting, cycling and weight-lifting are just a few other different disciplines that put extra stress on the upper back. In some individuals this could further lead to irritation of the sympathetic nervous system, resulting in the development of ME/CFS.

As I have said, ME/CFS patients are diagnosed primarily by the exclusion of other, better understood diseases. But it is perfectly possible, and common, for people to suffer from more than one disease or disorder at one time. This is why my discovery of physical signs that are common to ME/CFS and FMS patients is so important, and they provide a much-needed aid in the diagnostic procedure as shown in the previous chapter.

The Perrin Technique is primarily an osteopathic technique. Many of you reading this book may be more familiar with ME/CFS and FMS than with osteopathy. By now you may have a clearer understanding of the biophysical processes leading to ME/CFS and FMS, but you may still be wondering how osteopathy can help.

How osteopathy helps

One of the major concepts of osteopathy is that the structure of the body governs the function of the organs within. Osteopaths work on the principle that a patient's history of illnesses and physical traumas is written into the body's structure. It is the osteopath's developed palpatory sense that enables the practitioner manually to diagnose while treating the patient. The osteopath's job is to restore a healthy structure to the body and thus its function. The osteopath gently applies manual techniques of massage and manipulation to encourage movement of the bodily fluids, eliminate dysfunction in the motion of the tissues, relax muscular tension and release compressed bones and joints. The areas being treated require proper positioning to assist the body's ability to regain normal tissue function. One of the key principles of osteopathy laid down by its founder, Dr Andrew Taylor Still (1828–1917), is that illness is mainly due to stagnation of body fluids and that if you can stimulate blood flow and other fluid motion, including cerebrospinal fluid and lymphatic drainage, then the body will recover.

One of AT Still's students, William Garner Sutherland (already mentioned on page 44), noticed that when the bones of a dis-articulated skull were viewed in a certain way, they resembled the gills of a fish. Accordingly, he hypothesised, in 1898, that their shape was designed to allow for movement and so cranial osteopathy was born. By gentle pressure on the head one can help this movement aid the lymphatic drainage of the brain; as Sutherland said, 'When you tap the waters of the brain see what happens in the lymphatic system.'

Lubrication for effleurage

Congested and varicose lymphatics throughout the body are relieved by 'effleurage', a method of massage that requires stroking motions along the surface of the head, neck and trunk. To avoid any friction, which will aggravate any inflammatory condition, practitioners and patients must use plenty of lubrication when carrying out the effleurage. The type of oil or cream is very important. It should be hypo-allergenic and unscented. The oils that I use are coconut oil and sweet almond oil, although some practitioners prefer using an aqueous cream. Baby oil is not suitable, as it is a perfumed mineral oil, a by-product of refining crude oil to make gasoline and other petroleum products.

The concertina and siphon effects

The main focus of the treatment is to massage the lymph always in the direction towards the collar bones in a technique that I call the 'concertina effect'. As in a concertina or an accordion, where putting pressure on the ends of the bellows forces air through the instrument to produce the desired musical effect, so effleurage performed towards either clavicle (collarbone) on both sides creates a pressure that forces the lymph to drain out through the central drainage system into the subclavian veins (see Figure 4, page 10). This increased pressure of lymphatic fluid produced within the lymphatic ducts creates a negative pressure in the lymphatic vessels above and below, which then produces what is known as the 'siphon effect' which is familiar to anyone who has ever cleaned out the bottom of a fish tank – sucking on a tube creates a pressure gradient. Fluid will always flow from an area under higher pressure to an area of lower pressure. So, lymph will continue to drain from the entire system, eventually including the lymphatic system of the brain and spinal cord. Toxins stuck in the central nervous system, some for many years, will slowly and surely drain away after being sucked up, just like the siphon tube in the fish tank, into the main trunks and ducts of the lymphatic system.

The osteopathic techniques that I have developed to treat ME/CFS and fibromyalgia syndrome (FMS) patients are based on some new procedures that I have developed but mainly on standard procedures used by many trained osteopathic practitioners and some physiotherapists and chiropractors[1,2].

Reducing inflammation

The first task is to reduce any possible inflammation present at the damaged segments of the spine. This can be achieved in various ways. Some practitioners would prescribe anti-inflammatory drugs. However, contrast bathing (warm alternating with cold) is deemed preferable, as it has no toxic side effects. The warm compress usually consists of a warm (not hot) water bottle. Too hot a compress could scald the patient's skin. The 'cold' is as cold as the patient can tolerate and this is sometimes just cool, i.e. fridge temperature; it is safer if a frozen pack is wrapped with a cover, especially as ME/CFS patients often cannot tolerate extremes of temperature. Frozen peas, which easily mould around the back, can be a used, although special cold compress packs, which remain soft even when frozen, are preferable and less messy, especially if the peas fall out of the bag!

My clinical experience has shown that the sequence of contrast bathing that gives the best results in reducing the inflammation in ME/CFS is as follows:

COLD –	3 minutes	}
WARM –	1 minute	}
COLD –	1 minute	} Total 10 minutes
WARM –	1 minute	}
COLD –	1 minute	}
WARM –	3 minutes	}

This process has no adverse side effects, and so it is safe to be used as many times as required. Application of at least three times a day to the upper thoracic region is recommended if there is inflammation in the neck and shoulders (or there are cerebral symptoms) and the lower thoracic area when the abdominal or lower extremities are affected. The main advantage of contrast bathing over anti-inflammatory drugs is that it works quickly and directly on the affected area. Even when there is no palpable or visible inflammation, shown by heat and redness, contrast bathing to improve circulation in the thoracic region is still advised as it will aid circulation in the region which will, in turn, help the lymphatic drainage of the spine and help improve the health of the tissue lying alongside the spine.

With FMS, patients respond better to cold only on the spine for 5 minutes followed by, or at the same time, placing warm compresses or a warm water bottle on the surrounding muscles. For example, if there is much pain in the shoulders, arms and hands then the patient should apply warm to these areas and the cold (not freezing) compress on the very bottom of the neck and upper back.

Likewise, if the pain is in the legs and feet, then warm these areas and at the same time place cool packs on the upper lumbar spine, around the waist level. This is the level supplying the bottom of the sympathetic nerve chains mentioned earlier and will hopefully reduce the overstimulation of the sympathetic nerves of the abdomen, legs and feet.

Perrin Technique protocol for fibromyalgia syndrome (FMS)

Note that the treatment of FMS is virtually the same as with ME/CFS with two exceptions. I advise far less effleurage (stroking massage, explained below) as most patients with FMS can only cope with a little effleurage before the skin becomes painful. It is essential with FMS to use more oil or cream to avoid any friction. Leon Chaitow, ND, DO (1937–2018), a world-renowned author and practising naturopath, osteopath, and acupuncturist, advocated more long-lever stretches for fibromyalgia, which I have found to be most useful. So, with FMS

I reduce the effleurage and gently stretch the spine with the long-lever technique mentioned below.

The other major difference between the treatment of ME/CFS and of FMS is that although I always advise against over-treating with ME/CFS, I am doubly cautious with FMS concerning the whole treatment session. Besides effleurage that should be minimal, the use of direct manipulation, and high velocity-low amplitude manipulation should be restricted to the bare minimum in FMS.

Post-traumatic FMS

The condition known as post-traumatic fibromyalgia, which is a very severe form of fibromyalgia that occurs as a result of a traumatic injury, usually to the neck, such as a whiplash injury sustained in a car crash, remains very difficult to treat. I have found in these cases that the most gentle cranial stimulation, together with a multi-discipline approach such as hypnosis, mindfulness, or psychotherapy to advise on coping strategies plus acupuncture may help. Sometimes the pain is too much for even the slightest touch, and then I have to hope there will be some improvement from the other approaches before I can try and help.

A physician who suffered from this disease was Dr Mark Pellegrino, who shares the theory of fibromyalgia researchers such as Dr Muhammad B Yunus, at the University of Illinois College of Medicine. They maintain that the disease bears all the hallmarks of hypersensitisation of the central nervous system together with neuro-hormonal dysfunction, as seen in ME/CFS due to hypothalamic and sympathetic nervous system overload.

Chapter 5

The 10 steps of the Perrin Technique

The manual treatment of each ME/CFS patient (preferably performed by a licensed Perrin Practitioner) consists of the following 10 stages (explained in detail in Chapter 10 of *The Perrin Technique 2nd Edition*):

1. Effleurage to aid drainage in the breast tissue lymphatics
2. Effleurage to aid drainage in the cervical lymphatic vessels
3. Gentle articulation of the thoracic region and soft tissue techniques with upward effleurage
4. Effleurage to aid drainage in the cervical lymphatic vessels
5. Soft tissue massage to relax muscles and encourage lymph drainage of the cervicothoracic region
6. Further cervical effleurage towards the subclavian region
7. Functional and inhibition techniques to the suboccipital region
8. Further cervical effleurage towards the subclavian region
9. Stimulation of the cranio-sacral rhythm by cranial and sacral techniques
10. Final cervical effleurage towards the subclavian region.

As Rudyard Kipling (1865–1936) once said: 'The cure for this ill is not to sit still.' Movement is an essential part of the healing process. So gentle exercises are prescribed to improve the quality of thoracic spine mobility and the coordination of the patient. The treatment schedule listed above is almost the same as the protocol followed throughout clinical trials that I and colleagues conducted in the years 1996–1997 and 2000–2001; these are discussed in detail in *The Perrin Technique 2nd Edition*. It has altered slightly over the years as I have found that certain techniques further improve the neuro-lymphatic drainage. The amount of time spent, and the pressure exerted on to the patient whilst using these techniques, depends on the physical state of the patient and on the symptom picture at that particular stage in their therapy. So, as always with ME/CFS and FMS, with every patient the techniques are distinct, and each individual treatment session is marginally different from the other consultations with the patient.

The exact nature, content, intensity and timing of each treatment is determined by the trained and experienced practitioner.

As one can see from the 10 steps of the treatment, besides the effleurage/massage techniques there are also manoeuvres that improve movement and functioning of the spine and cranial stimulation (which commences near the end of each consultation). This technique is the most important and powerful part of the treatment as it directly affects the fluctuating, slow-wave known as the cranial rhythmic impulse (CRI), which is, according to my hypothesis (as explained on page 45), the pulse of neuro-lymphatic drainage. Cranial techniques have been shown to be effective in helping all aspects of the patient's health. In this technique, the osteopath's hand is placed in two different positions, cradling the head laterally and antero-posteriorly. The cranial procedure involves very gentle pressure and minimal movements. Although to the observer, and indeed from the patient's point of view, cranial techniques may seem very gentle, they are extremely powerful and often produce major changes with only a little application.

There are more specialised cranial techniques that I sometimes use, and this is all about the individuality of the treatment, palpating the patient's specific needs at the time of each treatment, so the holds may vary at each treatment, regarding how long and how much pressure one uses. Generally, it is very gentle, with the patient feeling very little going on until the cranial treatment is over. Cranial techniques, however, should always be done after the previous eight stages of the technique listed above.

Some practitioners refer to the CRI as the cranio-sacral rhythm. This is due to the fact that the rhythm can be palpated easily at the sacrum at the base of the spine as the cerebrospinal fluid moves down the spine from the cranium to the sacrum and then turns back and up towards the brain. The practitioner can palpate and further stimulate the CRI at this level by cradling the sacral bones when the patient lies supine (face up).

After treatment

Immediately after treatment you may feel slightly giddy and possibly even nauseous. To avoid fainting or being too disorientated you should first lie on your side, gently swing your legs over the edge of the treatment table and slowly sit up from the side-lying position. You should then have a slight rest just sitting at the side of the treatment table with your feet on the floor for a minimum of 10 seconds before trying to get up from the treatment plinth.

Sometimes it may be a few minutes before the patient can stand up following their treatment session, and some need a drink of water to help their nausea and dizziness. This is due to the fact that this treatment 'does what it says on the tin'. Real poisons/toxins are being released from the central nervous system during the half hour or so of the treatment session. The body has to be able to cope and we help the detox programme with a few choice supplements that should relieve many of the nasty side effects of this process. As the French artist Paul Cézanne and the animated character Shrek famously said, 'Better out than in'. However, another adage, 'Less is more', originally from a poem by Robert Browning and made famous by architect Ludwig Miles van der Rohe, encompasses my golden rule for treatment of ME/CFS and FMS. When doing the Perrin Technique, always apply this rule, especially concerning cranio-sacral treatment. Particularly in the early stages of treatment, care should be taken not to over-stimulate the drainage, especially the cranial rhythm, with too long or forceful a treatment as one might drain off excess toxins at one session, causing too much of a severe reaction. As the therapeutic programme progresses and the patient improves, the practitioner can gradually increase the intensity of treatment and, if necessary, use additional techniques.

Self-help advice

Osteopathic treatment is not synonymous with manipulation. Many treatments of numerous conditions would be found to be insufficient if they relied on manual therapy alone. As in standard osteopathic practice, advice is given to the patient to help improve their general health. Over the years, it is the patients who have followed my instructions to the letter who have done the best with the Perrin Technique.

I do realise that exercises and advice are not always easy to follow, but patients should try their best and hopefully see the benefit of being strict with the regime. The golden rule regarding exercises for ME/CFS and FMS is the same as with the treatment:

'PAIN = NO GAIN'.

You are doing nobody any favours if you push yourself through the pain barrier. Pain is the body's natural protection, telling you to stop and not to push on, especially as the pain control mechanisms of the brain in the basal ganglia and thalamus are disturbed in ME/CFS and especially in FMS. This leads to a reduction in the amount of the pain-suppressing neurotransmitter GABA and increased production of the pain stimulant neuropeptide P, which have both been shown to be disturbed when the neuro-lymphatic system becomes dysfunctional.

The most important advice, which is accepted by most experts in ME/CFS, is that of pacing. In 1989 when doctors were generally telling ME patients to exercise more, I advised patients to pace. I explain pacing by what I call 'the half rule' – that is, whatever the activity, whether walking, having a conversation or watching TV, always do half of what you feel capable of. In other words, when you do any physical or mental activity, always ask yourself, 'Can I do double without any problems afterwards?' If the answer is **no** or **maybe**, then you are doing too much. The answer to that question always has to be an unequivocal **YES**. Pacing reduces the strain on your sympathetic nervous system, which is paramount for improvement in your health. Without pacing there won't be any long-term benefit from any treatment of ME/CFS and FMS.

As the treatment improves your health, then gradually increase activity to recondition your body and improve your stamina. However, always stay within the half rule … as I always tell my patients: 'Half of more is still more'.

Chapter 5

As explained earlier in this chapter, manual treatment improves the function of the thorax and the spine. This is especially so when enhanced by routine mobility exercises. Some effective exercises to improve and maintain the quality of movement of the dorsal spine areas follow. I have described them in easy-to-understand English in the second person as these instructions are important for patients to follow as accurately as possible. (Thanks to Dr Lisa Riste for helping with the plain-language version.)

Dorsal rotation and shrugging exercises

Sitting down (see Figure 14), facing ahead, place your hands around both sides of your neck with thumbs nearest your shoulders, elbows facing forward and down. Slowly rotate your upper body, first to the right (from the waist up) keeping your head and neck facing the same direction as your upper body. This gentle rotation is designed not to stretch muscles and joints, but gradually and subtly to increase movement of your upper back. You should only rotate or twist about 45 degrees in total from right to left. Now twist gently and slowly, without stopping in the middle, to the left side. The movement must be rhythmic and as relaxed as possible during the entire process. This should be repeated five times each way.

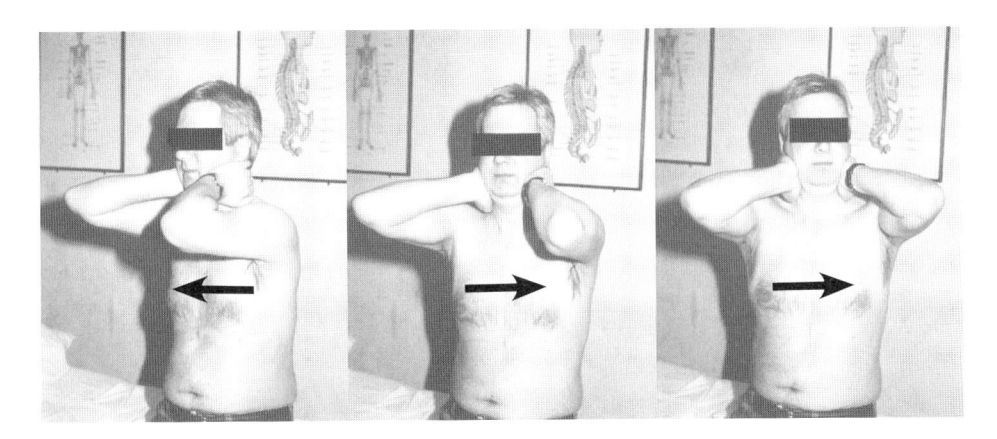

Fig. 14 Upper thoracic rotation exercise.

The Perrin Technique

In the next exercise (see Figure 15), while sitting, cross your arms and hug your shoulders with your hands. Then rotate your back five times each way through an arc of 45 degrees. Make sure that your head, neck and shoulders all stay in line with each other. This exercise encourages movement in the middle section of the thoracic spine.

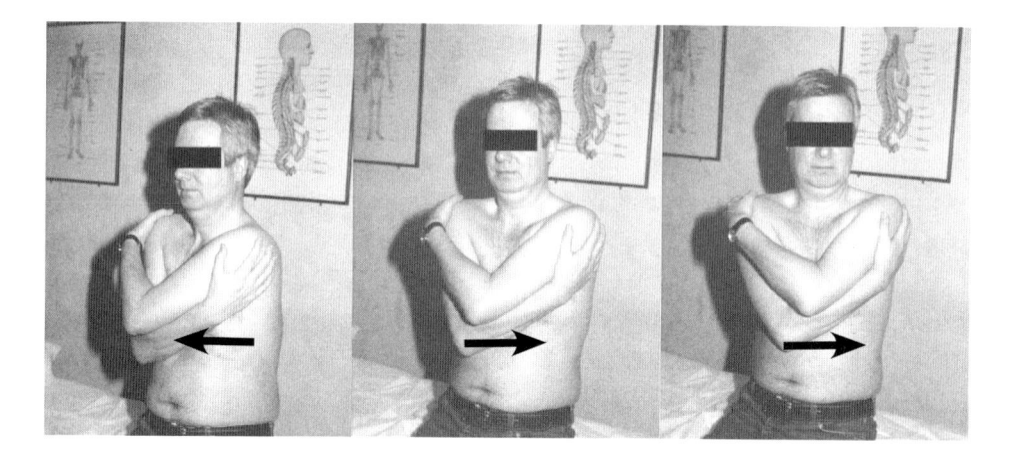

Fig. 15 Mid-thoracic rotation exercise

Finally, in the third exercise (see Figure 16), still sitting, fold your arms at your waist. Slowly rotate your back five times each way, again keeping your head, neck and shoulders in line. This exercise improves mobility of the lower thoracic spine.

Following the above three exercises, stand up if you are able, and gently roll your shoulders slowly forward five times and then slowly backwards, repeating the rolls five times (see Fig. 17).

The three-stage trunk rotations together with shoulder rolls will take about one minute, if done at the correct speed.

Chapter 5

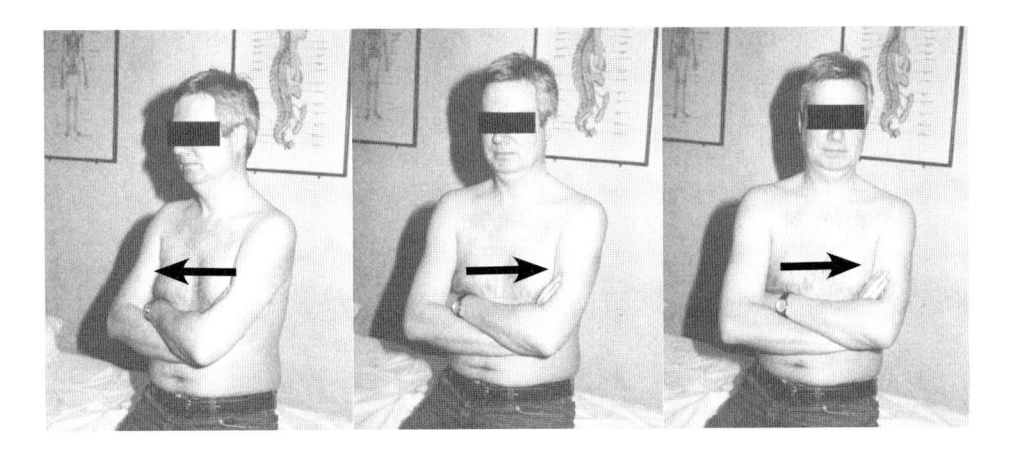

Fig. 16 Lower thoracic rotation exercise

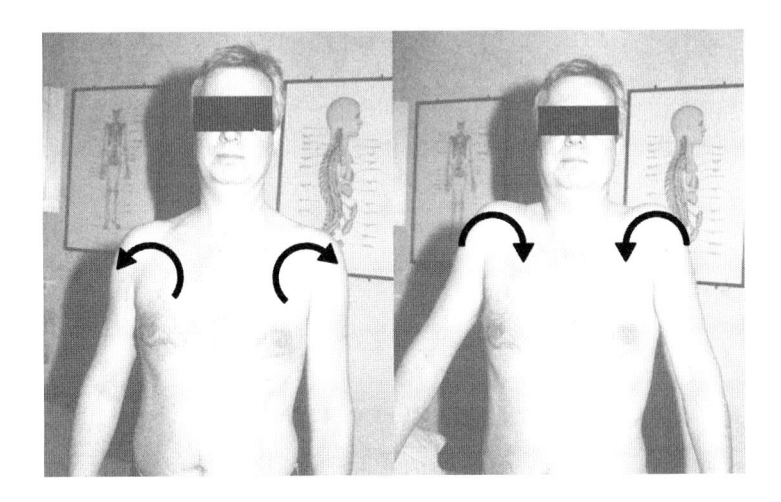

Fig. 17 Shoulder rolling exercise

You should carry out the entire sequence of rotation and shoulder rolling three times a day. Since it is a very gentle exercise, even if your ME/CFS is severe, this should not prevent you from carrying out these exercises. However, you are advised to cease exercises if pain develops at any time during or following the routine.

Cross-crawl

One can stimulate both halves of the brain to work together in harmony with the whole body by the following simple exercise, known as the cross-crawl. The cross-crawl exercise is basically marching on the spot crossing one limb over to the opposite side. The marching action should be slow and deliberate, with your right arm moving in unison with your left leg, with best results touching your flexed left knee with your right hand.

This action is repeated moving your left arm forward together with your right leg, touching your right knee with your left hand. ME/CFS patients sometimes find this simple task difficult to perform at the beginning of therapy, since their bodies are so un-coordinated. It is very important not to move the arm and leg of the same side together, as this will succeed in throwing your body (and mind) further out of balance.

After practising for a while, patients are able to carry out the cross-crawl exercise without too much difficulty. The marching routine is to be done for up to five minutes during an entire day, a minute or so at a time. Remember that it shouldn't exhaust you as any exercises that over-exert you will worsen your condition and are always to be avoided.

This technique can be adapted by very severe patients who are wheelchair-bound or even bed-ridden. This can take the form of the patient gently moving their left hand slowly up and down together with their right foot followed by their right hand together with their left foot, and flexing and extending each hand and foot five times at a time. This can be repeated every day, or more frequently if the patient feels that they are still following the half rule without ever exhausting themselves.

Strengthening exercises for hypermobile spinal joints

Sub-occipital hypermobility

If patients suffer from sub-occipital hypermobility/cranio-cervical instability, I

Chapter 5

advise the following isometric exercise routine (i.e. with only pressure but no actual movement). It is essential that no movement of the neck takes place. Repeat the six different stages of the exercises five to 10 times as long as it is not too taxing for you. The whole routine (below) should be completed three times a day as long as you can cope with the exercises and feel that it is not too strenuous. In other words, keeping with the tenet of the half rule, you should feel that you are easily able to do double the amount of exercise without aggravating your symptoms.

1. Lying down or sitting upright, gently hold one or both hands on your forehead. Try to slightly flex your neck, i.e. face looking downwards, but stop any movement with your hands pressed on your forehead so that your head remains at all times facing forward. This attempt to bend your head downwards should be maintained for three seconds and then you should gently relax the pressure before repeating the exercise five to 10 times in total (see Figure 18a).

2. Next try to slightly extend your neck (i.e. bending head back), again without any actual movement, stopping the extension with your hands pressed on the back of your head (occiput). This attempt to bend your head backwards should be maintained for three seconds and then you should gently relax the pressure before repeating the exercise five to 10 times in total (see Figure 18b).

3. Try to slightly tilt your head to the right, stopping any movement with your right hand on the side of your head. This attempt to bend your head sideways should be maintained for three seconds and then you should gently relax the pressure before repeating the exercise five to 10 times in total (see Figure 19a).

4. Repeat the same exercise in stage 3 for the left side (see Figure 19b).

Note: The white arrows in Figures 18-20 represent the direction of resistance offered by your hands.

The Perrin Technique

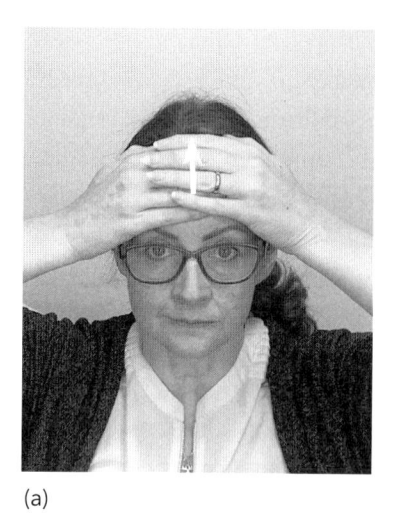

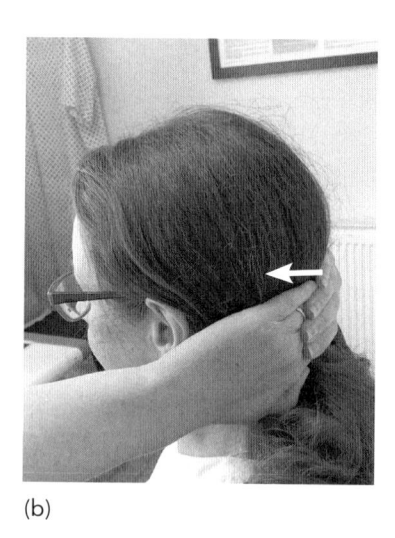

(a)   (b)

Fig. 18 Cervical isometrics: (a) Attempting to bend head forward, prevented by gentle backwards pressure of hands. (b) Attempting to bend head back, prevented by gentle forward pressure of hands.

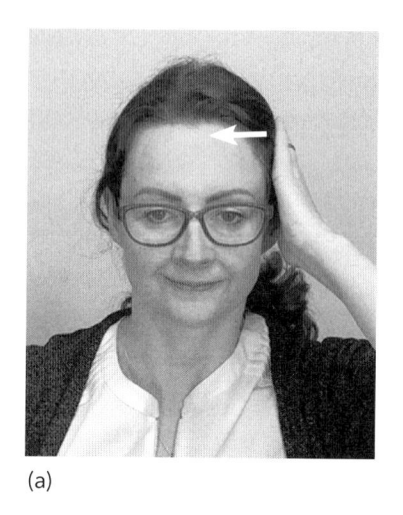

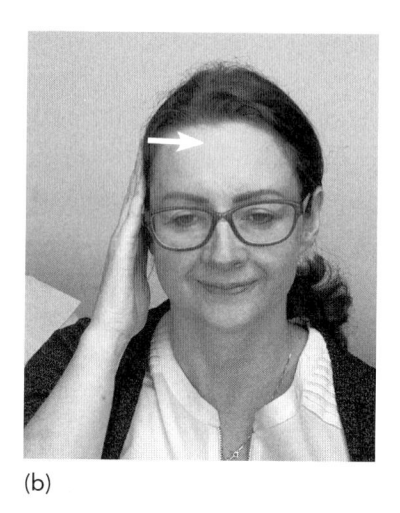

(a)   (b)

Fig. 19 Cervical isometrics: (a) Attempting to bend head to the left, prevented by gentle counter-pressure of left hand. (b) Attempting to bend head to the right, prevented by gentle counter-pressure of right hand.

Chapter 5

The first four stages gently strengthen the whole neck; however, the next two exercises are specifically designed to remedy the sub-occipital instability.

5. Now try to slightly flex the very top of your neck by trying to tuck in your chin, stopping any movement with both your thumbs pressed into the inside of your chin. This attempt to tuck in your chin should be maintained for three seconds and then you should gently relax the pressure before repeating the exercise five to 10 times in total. For the exercise to be successful it is important that little or no movement of your chin or neck takes place (see Figure 20a).

6. Try to slightly extend the very top of your neck by trying to poke out your chin, stopping any movement with one or both hands pressed against the front of your jaw (see Figure 20b). This attempt to push out your chin should be maintained for three seconds and then you should gently relax the pressure before repeating the exercise again five to 10 times in total. As with stage 5, it is essential that little or no movement of your chin or neck takes place.

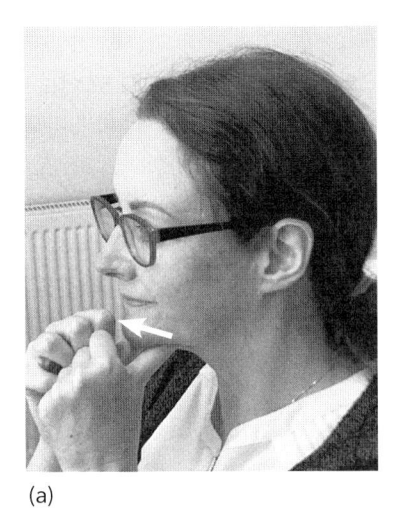

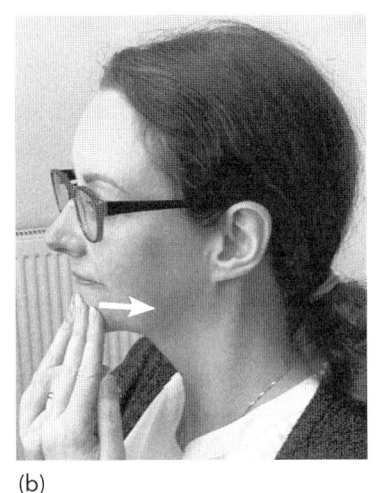

(a)   (b)

Fig. 20 Cervical isometrics: (a) Attempting to tuck in chin, prevented by gentle forward counter-pressure of thumbs. (b) Attempting to push chin forward, prevented by gentle backwards counter-pressure of fingers.

Hypermobility of the lower lumbar region

In cases of hypermobility of the lower lumbar region, I advise patients to carry out the following exercise routine. You should repeat the different stages of the exercises up to 10 times, three times a day, as long as it is not too taxing for you.

1. First, lie on your back, preferably on a firm surface such as a yoga mat, with knees bent. Lying on the bed will be okay if you find it difficult to lie on the floor.
2. Next, lift your bottom and lower back gently up a few centimetres from the floor and hold for three seconds.
3. Slowly lower your bottom and gently relax the muscles before repeating the exercise. For those familiar with yoga, this exercise is similar to 'the bridge' position but without lifting the bottom so high.

Home-massage routine

Patients are advised to aid the lymphatic drainage of their head and spine through a self-massage routine carried out at home which further aids lymphatic drainage from the central nervous system into the blood. As we now know, the main bulk of toxins are drained from the brain into the lymphatics during deep delta-wave sleep (see Chapter 1, page 13) which is why it is so restorative. However, we now know that ME/CFS and FMS patients unfortunately don't get much delta-wave sleep but too much alpha-wave sleep, which is non-restorative and leads to hyperarousal of the sympathetic nervous system in the brain.

Therefore, stimulating neuro-lymphatic drainage at night will hopefully mimic what is meant to happen naturally and you will wake up more refreshed as the toxins drain out of your central nervous system. So, the full routine as shown below should be done once at night, preferably just before bedtime.

Nasal release

Sitting down, rest your elbows on a table in front of you and apply gentle pressure with the pads of both index fingers to just below where the upper and lower eyelids meet (in the corner of your eyes). Push slightly upwards or, if more comfortable, pull slightly downwards just above the bridge of your nose (see Figure 21). Choose the position that feels most comfortable and lets you breathe the easiest. If neither method is more effective at aiding breathing, then you should always choose downward pressure as the default method. For the first 10 days of this self-treatment, apply this pressure for seven minutes.

After the first 10 days, you should continue with nasal release for a one-minute period each day in order to maintain the improvement.

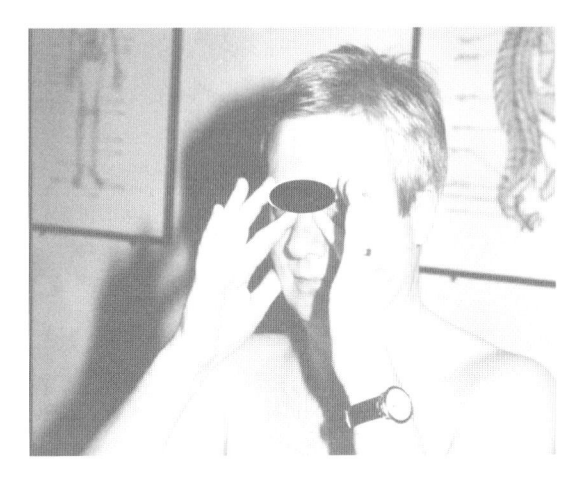

Fig. 21 Nasal release.

Facial massage

Spread the fingers of one hand across your face, as if trying to span your forehead, and slowly stroke your fingertips down your face to your chin (see Figure 22). Repeat this gentle facial stroking for 20 seconds with one downwards stroke roughly every four seconds.

The Perrin Technique

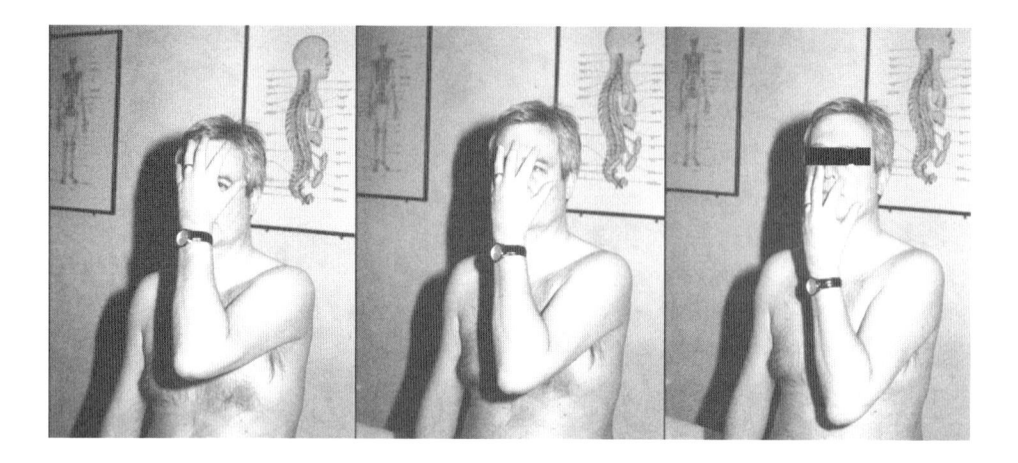

Fig. 22 Facial self-massage.

Head massage

You should now gently massage the sides and back of your head:

1. For the sides of your head: repeat the strokes used in the facial massage above, using your hands to gently stroke downwards on both sides of your head at once, from the top of your head to your chin, with the same slow rhythm again for 20 seconds (see Figure 23).
2. For the back of your head, repeat again with gentle downward stroking using both hands at the back of your head working down to your neck for a further 20 seconds.

For the remainder of the self-massage, you should use some massage oil. As I said earlier (page 53), this can be sweet almond oil, coconut oil or similar depending on any allergies or sensitivities you may have. NB: Avoid baby oil or any other petrochemical-based cream.

Chapter 5

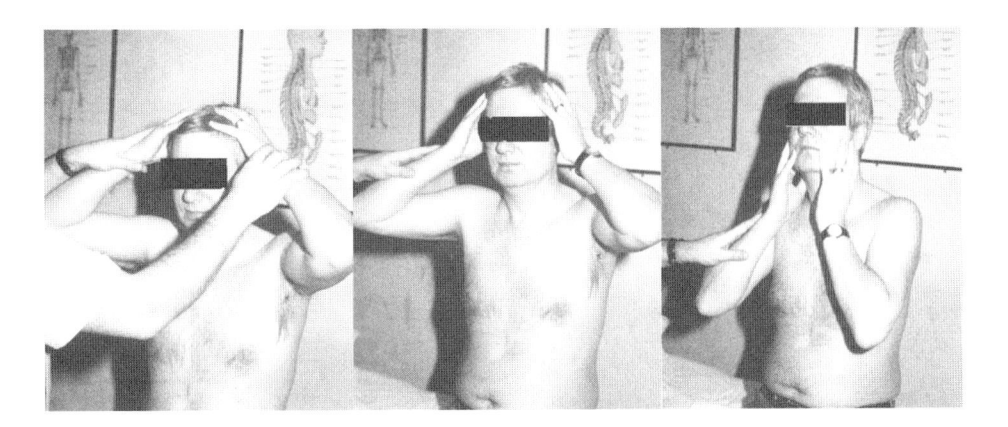

Fig. 23 Self-massage to head.

Self-massage to front of neck

Lie down and, using the oil, massage gently from the top of your neck just under your ear, down towards your collarbone using the back of your fingertips for 20 seconds on each side (see Figure 24).

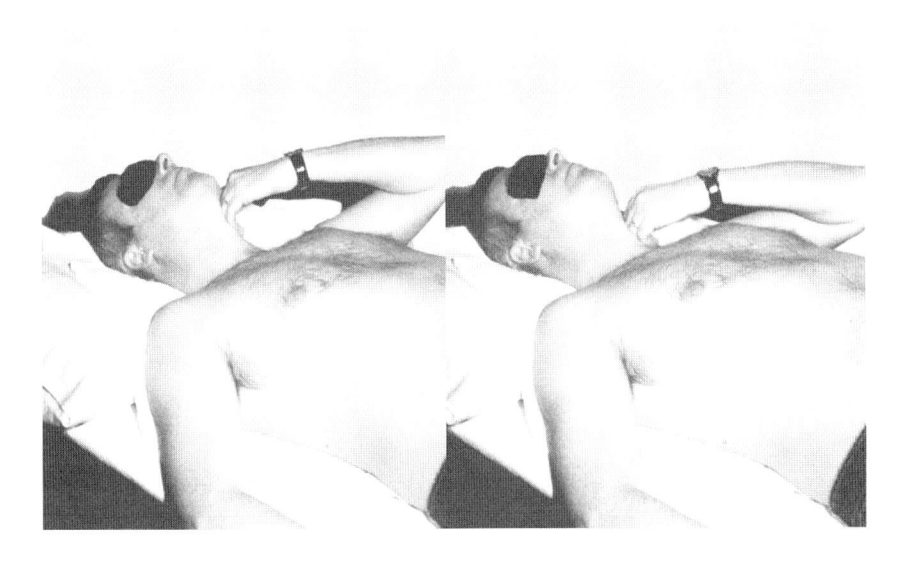

Fig. 24 Self-massage to front of neck.

Breast massage

The breast/chest massage is easiest done in three sections (outer, centre and inner), using massage oil, for 20 seconds in each area so the right and left areas are massaged for one minute each. The massage must always be towards the clavicles, thus directing the lymph away from the axillary (armpit) lymph nodes to avoid risk of glandular swelling in the armpits (see Figure 25).

Outer: Massage the side of your chest with a slow rhythmic stroking movement, with the flat fingertips of one hand and rubbing upwards with the other hand in a loose fist position. Start just underneath the breast area and work upwards towards the collarbone (not towards armpits).

Centre: Repeat the massage movements but working over the centre of the breast so the massage is up over the nipple area, again up to the collarbone.

Inner: This is the same movement but using the backs of the fingers with both hands flat on the inside area of the chest.

In Figure 25, the black arrow shows the direction of the self-massage technique. The pressure applied by the patient should be much less than during a treatment session, concentrating only on the superficial lymphatics.

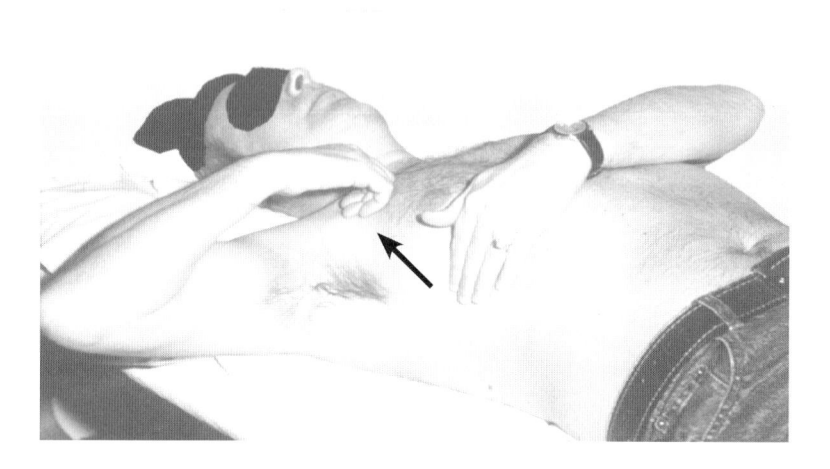

Fig. 25 Self-massage of the breast.

Chapter 5

Back massage

Having adopted a prone position, the patient receives back massage from a family member or friend. The massage routine comprises of one minute of gentle upward effleurage to the sides of the spine, finishing in the shoulder region, level with the clavicles. If no help is available, patients should use back brushes to accomplish the back massage. There are specific back massagers made out of wood with rubber heads, or other metal ones which are extendable and rubber rollers. Both these massage hammers are easy to use and are available to buy online. One useful tool to do the back massage for oneself is a small fluffy paint roller with a long handle used to paint behind wall radiators. Just move the roller upwards each side of the thoracic spine to the level of the collar bones just below the base of the neck.

Back of neck massage

The self-massage routine ends with slow downwards rhythmic massage of the back of the neck towards the level of collarbone carried out for 20 seconds on each side of the spine.

The full routine

The full routine is summarised in Table 5.1.

Table 5.1 The full routine. (To be completed at night, before bed, by the patient or with help from a carer.)

Nasal release	Rest elbows on table; place tips of index fingers on either side of nose (above the bridge); gently pull down/press up for 7 minutes for the first 10 days, followed by 1 minute thereafter
Facial massage	With fingers spread out apply a little pressure and gently stroke down the face for 20 seconds (five times taking 4 seconds each)

The Perrin Technique

Head massage	a. Gently stroke down the side of the head for 20 seconds each side
	b. Gently stroke down the back of the head for 20 seconds
Breast massage (use oil)	Up for one minute each side
	(NB Divide breast into three sections; outer, middle and inner and massage for 20 seconds each towards the collar bone and not the armpit)
Back massage (use oil)	Up for 1 minute each side of the spine (careful not to touch spinal column)
Neck massage – back (use oil)	Down for 20 seconds each side (simultaneously or one and then the other, whichever you find best)

Some patients whose symptoms are not too severe may find that a more regular self-massage routine speeds up the healing process. In the following extra top-up routine, only the head and neck are targeted, and it starts with the nasal release for only 1 minute. The shorter self-massage routine is completed with downward massage of the face and head followed by gently stroking down the front and back of the neck. This can be done anywhere as it is achieved without oil and without having to remove any clothing (see Table 5.2).

Table 5.2 The head and neck drainage routine
(To be completed up to three times a day)

Nasal release	For 1 minute
Facial massage	Down for 20 seconds at a time
Head massage	Down for 20 seconds at a time
Neck massage	Down for 20 seconds at a time each side, front and back

Active head rest

This is a do-it-yourself technique that I recommend for patients if I feel that the cranial flow could do with a little extra help, usually in the later stages of the treatment programme, as initially it may be too much too soon. It should only be done by patients at the beginning of therapy if they cannot access the actual Perrin Technique treatment. It is a simple exercise that is also taught by practitioners of the Alexander technique.

In the early days of osteopathy in the late nineteenth century, Dr Andrew Taylor Still, the founder of osteopathy, developed a similar exercise when he suffered from a severe headache. The story goes that he lay down and balanced his head on a swing. In those days in Missouri standing swings that rested just above the ground were all the rage, and Taylor Still found that by positioning his head at a certain angle he felt comfortable and in a short time his headache disappeared. This probably was the first cranial treatment ever performed.

One of the principles taught to me as a student osteopath was 'comfort governs function', which basically means that if the body is in the most comfortable position it will function better. So, if the head is positioned in the most comfortable position then the cranial flow, AKA the neuro-lymphatic drainage from the brain, will improve. Nowadays we don't use planks of wood or swings. You, the patient, should experiment with a paperback book or books placed under your occiput, which is the bone at the back of the head, until the most comfortable angle is achieved (see Figure 26). You should lie on a yoga mat or a duvet placed on the floor, so the ground is firm but not too hard, in a semi-supine position (on your back with knees bent) for about 10–15 minutes at night, preferably after the self-massage routine summarised in Table 5.1, just before going to sleep.

If you do not find any suitable book that you feel comfortable with, then this exercise should not be carried out as it will probably worsen the condition. It only works if it feels comfortable … remember: 'comfort governs function'.

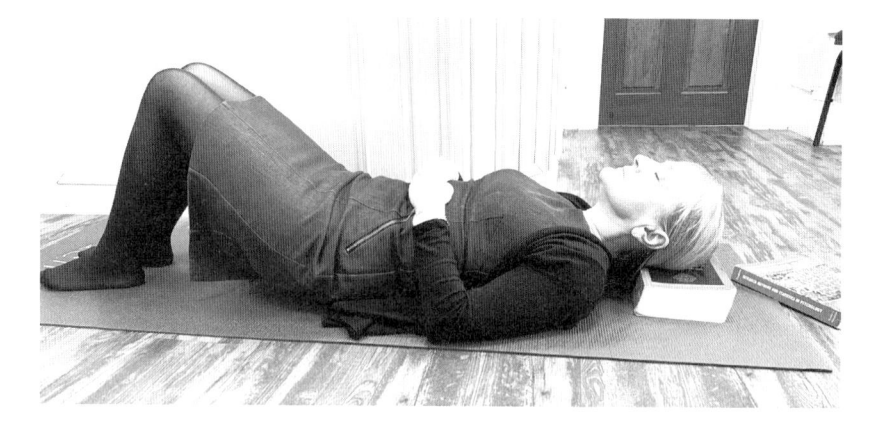

Fig. 26 Head rest exercise.

Returning to good health

Patients should try to avoid any stress, whether physical, mental or emotional, whenever possible. It isn't always easy and sometimes it's impossible, but you should try as hard as possible to reduce stress.

Activities that exert strain on the body are to be avoided. If your occupation involves too much physical or mental activity, you are advised to stop work temporarily or reduce your workload. This especially applies to tasks that put extra mechanical strain on your thoracic spine.

Physical and mental tasks that exert too much strain on you should, if possible, be done by a helpful colleague. Members of your family need to share the workload at home, including any paperwork, to make life as bearable as possible, until treatment has restored you to better health.

If you usually spend time in front of a computer, or VDU, or other device, or if you are desk-bound at work, you should stand up every half-hour for a minute or two and walk around the office. You should also take a 15-minute break, every two hours.

You should avoid slumping into a soft chair. When relaxing, you should sit in a supportive chair and if your ME/CFS or FMS is severe, aim to lie on your side as much as possible on a couch or a bed with your head well supported and a pillow between your knees. Lying on your side puts minimal strain on to your spine. It has also been shown that the neuro-lymphatic drainage occurs more when lying on the side and that a lateral sleeping position is the best position to most efficiently remove waste from the brain.

Diet and nutrition

In Chapter 5 of *The Perrin Technique 2nd Edition*, there is a comprehensive section on advice often given to ME/CFS and FMS patients by nutritionists and dietitians. Although there are specific needs for many patients with allergies and sensitivities, generally I advise most patients to vary their diet to provide as much diversity as possible. This reduces the possibility of placing strain on any particular region of the gastrointestinal system. All patients should reduce their intake of sugar and yeast, dairy products and foods containing gluten. Processed foods should be avoided as much as possible and brown flour and brown sugar should replace the white variety.

Stimulants such as caffeine are to be reduced and avoided altogether if possible. Decaffeinated coffee and decaffeinated tea or herbal tea can be drunk instead, but, because decaffeinated coffee has been shown to increase cholesterol levels, this should be taken only in moderation. Naturally caffeine-free tea such as Rooibos/Red Bush tea is preferable.

Patients should eat regular, healthy meals and drink plenty of healthy fluids, such as filtered or bottled mineral water – 2 litres a day for an adult should be enough.

I am totally against smoking as it has so many proven detrimental effects on health; however, the stress of trying to stop smoking may be too much for some patients and place excess strain on the sympathetic nervous system so, as much as I hate saying this, for some patients it is better to continue smoking than attempting to quit while they are trying to recover from ME/CFS and/or FMS.

Alcohol is an absolute NO! NO! for anyone with ME/CFS. This is for two fundamental reasons. The detrimental effects alcohol has on the liver are well documented and it is known that alcohol is the main cause of cirrhosis and liver disease. The main aim of the Perrin Technique is to drain toxins out of the central nervous system into the lymphatic system. The lymphatics will eventually drain the toxins into the bloodstream, with most ending up in the liver, which will need support rather than an extra further toxic load provided by alcohol.

However, the main reason why even a small amount of alcohol aggravates ME/CFS, and FMS, is due to its effect on the brain. We now know which are the main areas affected by a backflow of the neuro-lymphatics into the brain. Research has shown that when the drainage through the perivascular spaces is stopped there is a build-up of toxins in the thalamus and basal ganglia of the brain. The thalamus contains high levels of N-methyl-D-aspartate (NMDA). The methyl in the name is the clue, as this is the neurochemical affected when one drinks any alcohol and it is this neurotransmitter as well as GABA in the basal gonglia, that causes many of the symptoms of drunkenness. In ME/CFS and FMS, NMDA overstimulation leads to increased pain and more sleep disturbance as well as reduced cognitive function. So, alcohol, even a tiny drop, will usually worsen a patient's symptoms and, indeed, many patients find they cannot tolerate much alcohol anyway, with a small amount making them feel drunk.

This brings us to the next part of the advice to patients to aid their return to better health – supplements. Many supplements come in tinctures in little bottles which allow droplets of the remedy to be taken easily into the body rather than in pill or capsule form. The liquid medium of the tincture is usually alcohol-based and so if one takes tinctures of supplements with alcohol then drop them into boiling water first which will evaporate the alcohol, then wait until the water has cooled down before drinking the safe mixture.

Supplements

As well as a healthy diet, a supplement of vitamins C and B complex is advised. The former increases the patient's resistance to infection, while B complex improves energy production and general functioning of the nervous system. A daily dose of 500 mg of vitamin C and a strong, or whole, B complex tablet are recommended. Vitamins B and C are both water-soluble so that any excess is excreted from the body. However, one of the functions of vitamin C is to aid the absorption of calcium, so there is a risk of developing kidney stones if the vitamin C intake is too high. I always try to err to the side of caution and so advise patients to take only 500 mg a day.

Beware of taking so many different supplements that any possible benefit is likely to be outweighed by undesired side effects. In addition, many supplements can have an adverse reaction with other medications and may exert a strain on the gut as well as the liver and thus the lymphatics and the sympathetic nervous system. This will undoubtedly worsen the symptoms of ME/CFS and FMS.

One of my patients was taking so many supplements and prescribed medications that the first instruction I gave to her was to reduce all these supplements and go back to her doctor and check which medications she could stop or reduce the dose of (see Figure 27). It took quite a while for her body to pick up after

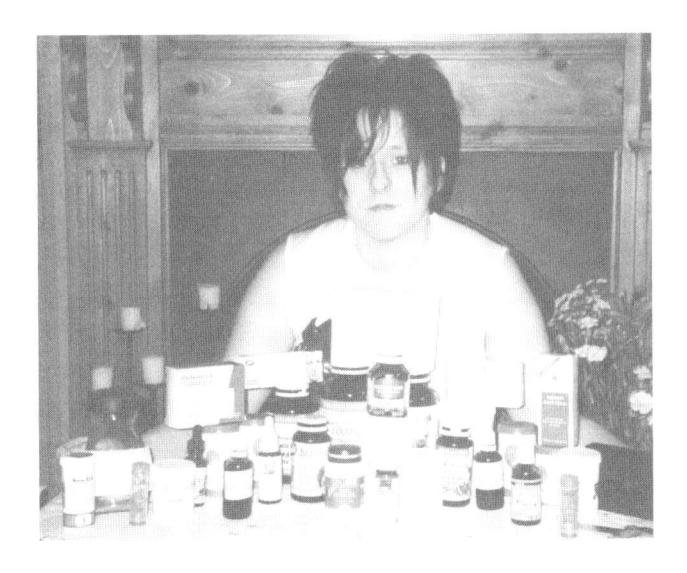

Fig. 27 An ME/CFS patient and her daily medication.

reducing this overload of supplementation and medication. However, together with the treatment she received from myself and one of my colleagues, she began to recover as is clearly demonstrated in the photo of her taken a few years on (see Figure 28). It is always best to seek expert professional advice when taking any medicinal treatments, whether pharmaceutical or herbal. So, speak to your doctor, pharmacist, naturopath, nutritionist or herbalist to find out what is best for you.

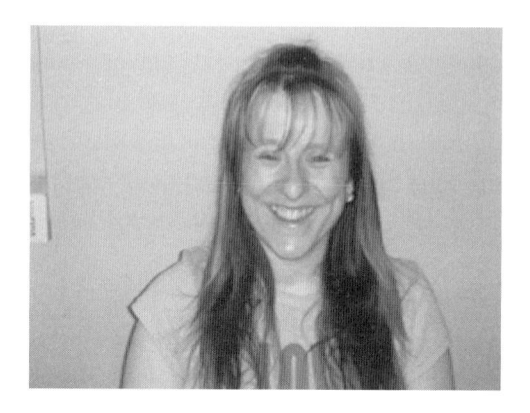

Fig. 28 The same patient after receiving the Perrin Technique and reducing her supplements and medication intake.

Even though excessive use is harmful, occasionally supplements may be needed. After a patient has received a good few treatments, and when the overall symptoms of ME/CFS or FMS start to lessen, many patients begin to develop a full-blown cold or suffer from flu for maybe the first time in years. This may sound crazy, but this is usually a very positive sign. It means that the immune system is starting to work properly after a very long period. In many cases of ME/CFS, initially there is an upward regulation of the immune response, so in the early stages, patients with ME/CFS rarely experience colds or flu, they just feel constantly ill with their general ME/CFS and FMS symptoms worsening. It is akin to a troop of marine commandos attacking a country which responds by dropping a nuclear bomb on the commandos, killing them but destroying a large part of the country in the process. The immune system of an ME/CFS patient will initially over-react to a virus, bacterium or fungus and kill the offending pathogen, but at the same time use up their energy reserve, exhausting the patient and aggravating all the other symptoms.

This overactive immune response has been demonstrated in recent research at King's College London. The research team demonstrated that in the early stages of the disease, the immune system is 'primed' to give exaggerated responses to infections which exhausts the patient and leads to chronic fatigue. However, this hyper-immunity didn't seem to last for more than six months. They concluded that in ME/CFS there is an abnormal immune mechanism.

Eventually, as the immune system starts to try and balance, there is more and more chance of developing colds and other infections, like normal individuals. However, some severely ill patients eventually suffer from a depleted immune system where the whole immune process has become exhausted. These very debilitated patients become susceptible to infection after infection which ultimately leads to disastrous effects on their overall health. In the very worst cases this eventually can cause organ or system failure. (See page 84 for supplements to boost the immune system in cases of infection and/or likely infection.)

Getting worse before getting better

One proof that the Perrin Technique is not a placebo is the fact that most patients feel a great deal worse at the beginning of their treatment. Placebo treatments generally do not make you feel worse. The reason for this initial exacerbation in the symptoms is that, for the first time, the toxins embedded (possibly for years) in the central nervous system are being released into the rest of the body.

Headaches and pain are due to excess toxicity. As the treatment encourages the toxins to leave the brain, they will initially affect the superficial tissues in the head and, as they drain down to the rest of the body, pain may follow. We know from the earlier studies of the glymphatic system by the research team at Rochester University in New York, that the first points of toxic build-up when the drainage stops are the thalamus and the basal ganglia, which control pain perception around the body. So, any pain felt by the patient due to stimulation of any nociceptor (pain receptor) outside the brain is exaggerated. However, the toxins within the brain do not cause actual pain since there are no nociceptors within the brain itself. Nevertheless, toxins do affect the *function* of the brain and spinal cord, and this accounts for most of the symptoms of ME/CFS and FMS.

Another unpleasant sign that occurs when the body's drainage is improving is the appearance of spots, boils and other skin eruptions. Until the lymphatic channels are working properly, the toxins have to go somewhere and the quickest way out of the body is often through the skin. These normally clear up as the treatment progresses. Some patients in the past have suffered from severe acne which occurs when the oil from sebaceous glands blocks hair follicles in the skin. Bacteria which infect the plugged follicles, causing the pustules seen in acne, may resurface with treatment and re-infect the hair follicles leading to a resurgence of the acne.

The first few weeks, or sometimes months in severe cases, are always the most trying for the patient. In clinic I have often noticed that the worse the patient is in the early stages of treatment, the better, usually, it bodes for their prognosis as the toxins flow out of the central nervous system. However, we need the patient to cope with the side effects and if the reaction is too unpleasant and the patient suffers too much, it can be counterproductive.

The Perrin Technique is patient-centred at all times. It is important that the practitioner listens to the patient and initially goes very softly, softly with the treatment. If the patient is in too much pain with the initial treatment, or other symptoms become unbearable, the practitioner should lessen the treatment intensity and sometimes space out the treatment sessions to a level where the patient can cope. Occasionally, patients respond better when the treatment is more intense and more frequent. As I have stressed throughout the book, every ME/CFS patient is different.

In the early days of my treatments, when I was developing my techniques, some patients dropped out of therapy as they could not cope with the side effects. I realised that every patient needs a different amount of treatment and, by listening

Chapter 5

to the symptoms of the patient at the early stages, both patient and practitioner can work out the routine that suits the patient's condition and achieve the best results in the longer term.

The main aspects for ME/CFS and FMS sufferers to focus upon are the changes occurring with the treatment. (If change has not occurred in any way during the first 12 weeks of treatment, the patient may have to take an alternative route in their search for a cure.) My treatment often hugely improves the patient's health, but most will need other treatments in tandem in order to alleviate all symptoms. I have noticed that other treatments – whether they be based on nutrition or pharmaceuticals – work better after the patient's neuro-lymphatic pathways have improved. Patients who have tried supplements before treatment, to no avail, are advised to try some of the supplements again after undergoing the Perrin Technique, as they may now prove more effective.

The jigsaw puzzle analogy

The Perrin Technique 2nd Edition includes (see its Chapter 5) many different approaches that can be used in conjunction with my treatment. The analogy I like to use to explain the importance of treating the neuro-lymphatic dysfunction in ME/CFS and FMS is that of a jigsaw puzzle.

When one tries to complete a jigsaw, it is best to start with the corners and edge pieces first. The four corners of the recovery jigsaw in ME/CFS and FMS are pacing, rest, relaxation and meditation/mindfulness. Pacing all physical and mental activities (the half rule), rest as much as you can and relax when resting if possible. If you cannot relax due to many stress factors in your life, then use meditation techniques such as mindfulness. The edge pieces are the treatment protocol that is the Perrin Technique, correcting the biomechanics and improving the neuro-lymphatic drainage and thus creating a framework for the rest of the picture to be filled in.

Sometimes the jigsaw puzzle of recovery is made up of only corners and edges, or just a few pieces in the middle, which makes the task much more straightforward

The Perrin Technique

and represents a patient making a complete recovery with just my standard advice and treatment.

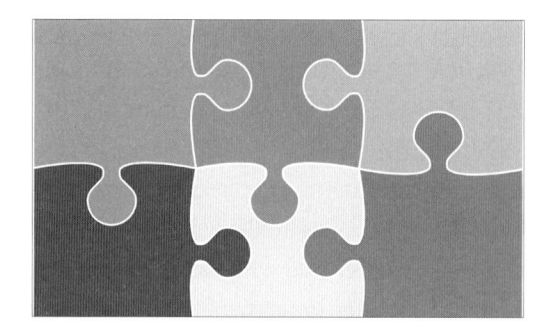

Fig. 29 Simple jigsaw puzzle of a few pieces, which is easy to solve.

Unfortunately, most cases are much more complex, with many difficult sections to be filled in. The supplements, medications, diets and talk therapies all form part of the sea and sky in the jigsaw puzzle picture of health.

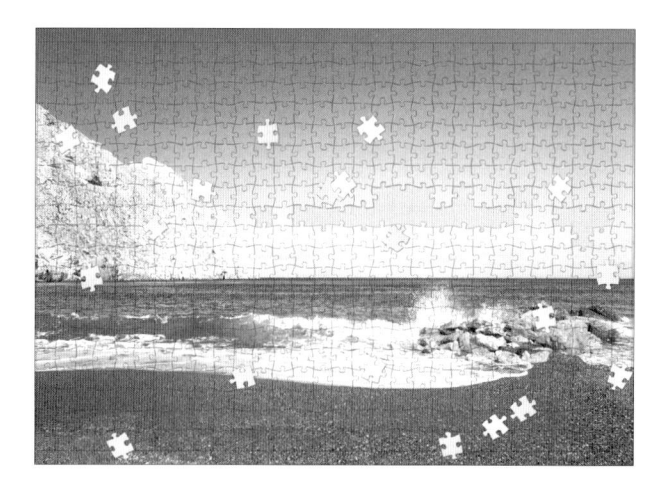

Fig. 30 Complex jigsaw puzzle with lots of sea and sky, making it very difficult to solve without the guidance of the corners and edges.

Chapter 5

One can of course start with the centre of a challenging jigsaw puzzle first, but it will make the task much more difficult and one could give up before the picture is complete.

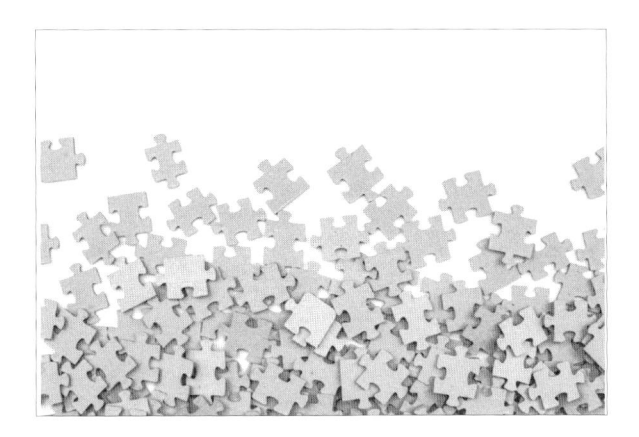

Fig. 31 A random approach to solving a jigsaw puzzle, without any clues.

Sometimes it seems too difficult and there are so many symptoms and problems that the practitioner doesn't know where to begin.

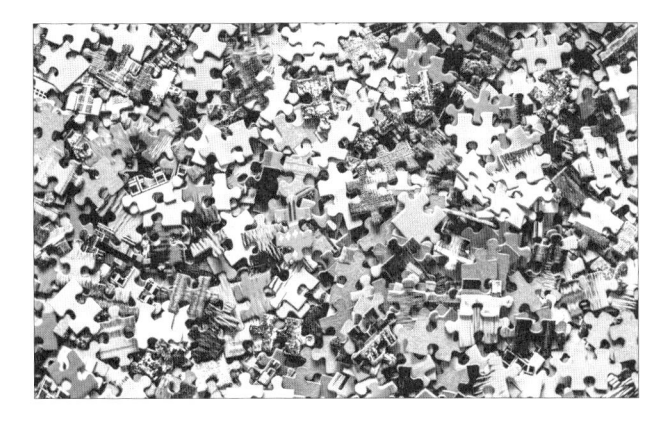

Fig. 32 An overwhelmingly complicated jigsaw puzzle representing a really complex case of ME/CFS or FMS.

So, start with the corners and edges to bring about the best result.

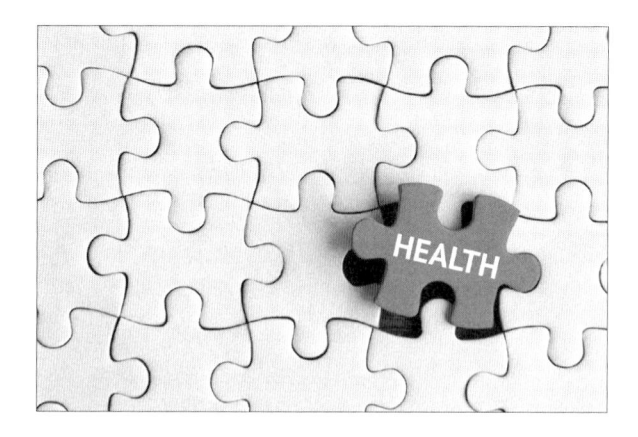

Fig. 33 Completing the puzzle with the corners and edges in place first.

For colds and flu

When patients do start to develop full-blown colds and other infections, some are really excited, as they remember me telling them in their initial consultation that this is sometimes a sign of the immune over-activation lessening and a good symptom. Some have come into the clinic with a big smile across their faces telling me with glee that they have had a proper cold complete with coughing, sneezing and red nose and it lasted a few days but they have mostly recovered without any major effect on their ME/CFS or FMS symptoms. However, we don't want the patient to continue with repetitive infections, so to help avoid the immune system going into free fall when infection strikes, I recommend a number of supplements to help.

- **Garlic** is known for its antimicrobial properties. I usually advise patients with infections to take the highest dose possible of allicin. This is one of the active ingredients of garlic and has been shown to exhibit antibacterial activity against a wide range of gram-negative and gram-positive bacteria, which won't directly help with viruses, but reduces the chance of secondary bacterial infection that could lead to pneumonia; allicin has also been shown to promote antifungal activity, particularly against *Candida albicans*, antiparasitic activity, including against some major human intestinal protozoan parasites, and antiviral activity.

- **Phytosterols** (plant sterols) have been shown to target specific lymphocytes – Th1 and Th2 cells – improving immune activity. I regularly advise patients to take a small dose of plant sterols as preventative supplements when there may be an outbreak of flu in their neighbourhood, and if they are suffering symptoms of colds and flu then the maximum dose helps balance the immune system as they fight off the infection.
- **Echinacea.** If the allicin and phytosterols don't help I would advise the patient to next try echinacea – a good natural immune system stimulant. Echinacea, also known as coneflower, is a native of central North America and used by native American tribes for sore throats, snake bites and sepsis. *Echinacea purpurea* is the most commonly used form. It seems to help the immune activity rather than target specific viruses. The recommended dose is usually in the region of 500 mg taken three times a day. However, echinacea shouldn't be used for more than a few weeks at a time and it is often recommended only for short-term use.
- One of nature's natural antibiotics, **bee propolis**, is also a useful tool when fighting infections.
- Another very effective, but probably the most hideous-tasting natural remedy, is **grapefruit seed extract** which enhances the immune system and can be used to help with all manner of infections, whether parasitic, viral, bacterial or fungal. Grapefruit seed extract has been shown to be effective at very low concentrations to reduce candida, and bacterial loads.

Flu jabs – and now covid jabs – are at the patient's discretion. Most stockpiled vaccines used to contain thimerosal (which is a mercury-based preservative). However, most flu vaccines are now made differently, so patients should be okay. It is still important to check with your doctor and pharmacist that the vaccine is toxin-free. Patients with heavy-metal poisoning struggle to respond to treatment since the heavy metals lie ingrained deep within the glial cells of the brain. Therefore, the standard lymph drainage techniques are simply not powerful enough to drain the heavy metals away. Detoxing with specific natural agents such as *Chlorella* or spirulina is necessary in these cases to help with the overall treatment process.

Frequency of treatment

At the beginning of treatment, it is important that the patient is treated once a week and that the treatment remains regular and weekly. This usually carries on for at least the first 12 weeks and, slowly, as the symptom picture improves, there is a gradual increase in the time between consultations. With very severe cases, weekly treatments may be necessary for much longer than three months.

Eventually, when patients remain symptom-free between their six-monthly check-ups and are able to perform all reasonable activities, doing all they could do before they were ill with no side effects, I will score them 10 out of 10. This is difficult to achieve, but it does happen every so often and is a wonderful feeling for both sufferer and practitioner. When I discharge the 10/10 patients it gives me the motivation and strength to carry on my clinical work treating some very severe bed-ridden patients and continue my research into ME/CFS and FMS.

While acknowledging that every patient is different, I have devised a chart (Table 5.3) based on the general severity of the illness that is a guide to both the patient and practitioner when calculating the overall prognosis.

Table 5.3 is a sliding scale and should be used as a general guide. In other words, if a patient initially scores 5/10 on ME/CFS alone, and is also suffering from another disorder, the overall score may be 4/10 or lower. If the physical findings during the examination are very evident and apparent, the overall score is lowered. As I have said, I often find that the patient is trying to appear healthier than they really are. This fits the profile of average ME/CFS sufferers who try as hard as they can to keep going until, eventually, they have to admit they cannot go on or they just collapse.

Table 5.3 The outlook

Score	Description	Prognosis
1	Extreme symptoms and signs for more than a year. Totally bed-ridden or sitting all day, little cranial flow palpable.	3 years +
2	Severe symptoms and signs for more than a year. Bed-ridden or sitting all day, little cranial flow palpable.	2 years+
3	Severe symptoms and signs for more than a year, resting most of the day, little cranial flow palpable.	2 years
4	Severe symptoms and signs for 6–12 months, resting most of the day, little cranial flow palpable.	18 months+
5	Severe symptoms and signs for at least 6 months; able to carry out light tasks but requires regular rest periods.	12–18 months
6	Moderate symptoms and signs for at least 6 months; able to work part-time with a struggle.	8–12 months
7	Moderate symptoms and signs for at least 6 months; able to work full-time with difficulty.	8 months
8	Moderate symptoms and signs for at least 6 months; daily life slightly limited. Symptoms worsen on activity.	6 months
9	No symptoms but still signs of slight lymphatic engorgement and experiences mild symptoms following over-exertion.	3 months
10	Symptom-free for at least 6 months. Able to live a full active life … within reason.	Discharged

Conclusion

As we can see, there is no 'one cap fits all' or 'magic bullet' approach to beating ME/CFS or FMS, as every individual patient has a unique set of symptoms due to the individuality of the condition, with myriads of different toxins affecting trillions of combinations of neurological pathways in the brain. The Perrin Technique offers a treatment and self-help programme that helps most, but isn't a cure-all approach. It involves a patient-practitioner partnership, where the treatment is always patient-centred but often takes time to see the benefit. Most patients with ME/CFS and FMS are helped by the Perrin Technique and some in a matter of weeks or months. These two similar conditions are chronic illnesses and can take years and a multidisciplinary approach to achieve the desired result.

However, as shown in this handbook and elaborated in *The Perrin Technique 2nd Edition*, stimulating a healthy lymphatic drainage of the brain is paramount in helping patients, leading to symptomatic relief and a better quality of life, with some achieving full recovery from ME/CFS and FMS plus possibly many other neurological disorders.

Case: Noel's story

From a young age I had always been really sporty, running my first 10k race at 11 and making the school basketball team, right up to studying sports science at university, where I participated in boxing, swimming, running, basketball and coaching the wheelchair basketball team. Even after starting a career in medical sales, I still maintained my passion to keep fit and compete. Especially in running; I always loved to run, and I loved to win.

It's hard to say when my health started to suffer. I'd always seemed to pick up a virus here and there. But as I worked in the health industry it wasn't too surprising. However, my busy work schedule seemed to be taking its toll and I was getting more and more tired and no amount of rest would improve things. I would still run, but recovery was taking longer and longer.

I'd been to the GP several times and they always steered the diagnosis towards either a nasty virus or depression. Unconvinced, I started to research possible illnesses and realised that ME appeared to describe the symptoms I'd been suffering. When I presented this to the GP I was told that it could well be ME, but that the waiting list for the ME or CFS clinic was nine months. In the meantime, I underwent a series of blood tests to rule out anything else.

I remembered that a friend of mine had suffered from ME many years before and had been treated effectively by an osteopath in Manchester.

At the first consultation Dr Perrin was absolutely convinced that I had ME. He rated me as quite severe, a 3 or 4 I think, on the scale of 1 to 10, despite my best efforts to appear perfectly well. Dr Perrin spelled out the course of treatment that would be required to get me back to a 10. He explained that it would get worse before it got better and that it would take two years. I admitted to my wife Laura, later at home, that I planned to be better in 18 months. Always competing!

Treatment began and the restrictions that I had to adhere to were difficult. There was very limited exercise and a new diet and supplements had to be adopted. Plus, a daily regime of hot and cold therapy and twice-daily lymphatic massages, lovingly provided by Laura. She became quite the expert and had my routine down to a fine art. I really couldn't have done it without her. She was my rock.

The first few treatments from Raymond were the worst as we would travel to Manchester for the therapy and then head back to Yorkshire. Laura would drive as on the return journey I would be almost comatose. The following day would be no better and I'd often be unable to get out of bed.

Slowly but surely over the coming months we progressed. Our daily routine was carried out with military precision. Our diets and lifestyles drastically changed – all in a bid to get me healthy again. Despite the recovery being gradual, there was a tipping point, around 12 months I think, when I started to feel much better. It was at this stage that I would quiz Dr Perrin about when I could start to run again. Raymond was very measured with his responses and encouraged me to be very careful. Walking at first and only doing half of what I thought I was able. As ever I was totally compliant, never pushing things too far, never wanting to risk a relapse.

After 18 months of treatment, Raymond signed me off. I can't explain the elation we felt at this point. We knew the treatment was working. However, to see the end result and feeling fully fit, back to myself again, was very special and we can't thank Raymond enough.

Noel Brennan, York, UK

Appendix 1

ME/CFS and FMS: Frequently asked questions

I have collected together here the questions I am most frequently asked. Many of the answers repeat information in earlier chapters, but I find it is worth presenting facts about ME/CFS and FMS in a variety of formats to allow the complexities of the conditions and their treatment to be fully understood. There is also new information, especially about the dos and don'ts during recovery, which I hope will be of immediate practical help.

What are the causes of ME/CFS and FMS?

There are many factors involved in the process leading to chronic fatigue syndrome/myalgic encephalomyelitis (ME/CFS) and fibromyalgia syndrome (FMS). The head may be traumatised at birth and this occurs more in first-born children as they are the first babies to pass through their mother's birth canal; alternatively, there may be a forceps or ventouse delivery, which places even more pressure on the baby's head. The first labour is usually the longest, but sometimes a very quick birth in younger siblings can also be traumatic for the small, vulnerable cranium of the newborn.

There may be a genetic predisposition affecting the normal development of the head or back and I see quite a few families with more than one member with ME/CFS and FMS. Years before the onset of symptoms, perhaps even in early childhood, the patient might have suffered from trauma to the head or spine. Teenage years bring with them problems of their own and the spine of a very active teenager is vulnerable to postural disturbance. The majority of ME/CFS and FMS patients were previously very sporty and/or high achieving people who pushed themselves to the very limit. However, there are a few sufferers who have tended to be 'couch potatoes' with a tendency to slouch and are more into reading and sedentary activities than sports during their teenage years but are still prone to developmental problems of the spine.

In the brain and spinal cord there is a fluid known as cerebrospinal fluid. One of the functions of the cerebrospinal fluid is drainage. Some poisons caused by infection, inflammation or toxins from a polluted environment (Chapter 3) enter the brain and spine and flow out through perforations in the skull and minute channels in the spine, entering the lymphatic system.

Certain structural problems affecting both the head and the spine together can result in no (or very little) drainage pathway for the cerebrospinal fluid to take (Figure 5, page 14). In someone with ME/CFS and/or FMS, these normal drainage points have initially become congested, leading to a build-up of poisons within the central nervous system.

The main organ in the brain to be affected by poisons is the hypothalamus, which is the control centre for the hormones and the sympathetic nervous system. The latter helps the body cope in times of stress. In ME/CFS and FMS, the toxic cocktail brewing in the hypothalamus leads to an overload of the sympathetic nervous system, which will have been affected by other stress factors – physical, allergic, emotional or infection – in the years leading up to the illness (Figure 6, page 14). One final trigger, which is usually a viral, bacterial or fungal infection, will lead to a breakdown in the normal functioning of the sympathetic nervous system.

Furthermore, the lymphatic system, which is meant to aid drainage, is under the control of the sympathetic nervous system. When this system is functioning poorly, toxins may be pumped in the reverse direction (Figure 12, page 42), which adds further poisons to the central nervous system. As the toxicity builds up, brain

Appendix 1

function worsens, leading to further sympathetic nerve disarray and increased toxicity in the brain and spinal cord. The vicious circle that ensues leads to the myriad of symptoms affecting the patient (see next). With ME/CFS and more so in FMS, the toxins affect the pain centres in the brain making the patient even more sensitive to any pain stimulus around the body.

What symptoms can you get with ME/CFS and FMS?

Below is an A-Z list of over 100 symptoms and common complaints that occur in these conditions. This list also appears in *The Perrin Technique 2nd Edition* (starting on page 369), with a short explanation as to the cause of each. Once interested parties, especially members of the healthcare professions, have read the *2nd Edition*, the symptoms of ME/CFS and FMS should no longer be a mystery. By understanding the mechanisms that cause these disorders one can logically explain all the varied symptoms listed. Over the years many patients have enquired whether a particular symptom is due to their illness: 'I started with this itching in my leg last week … could it be due to my fibromyalgia?' or 'I have been diagnosed with sleep apnoea and my GP doesn't know if this has anything to do with my ME.' Of course, there is always a possibility of another condition being present. In other words, you could be suffering from more than one condition and the symptom may be due to a completely different disease as well as the ME/CFS or FMS. As a general rule I would suspect the onset of a different disease if new symptoms seem to begin out of the blue and gradually worsen, when the major symptoms of the ME/CFS or FMS are responding well to treatment.

A

Acne

Allergies

Alopecia (hair loss)

Amenorrhoea (loss of periods)

Anosmia (loss of smell)

Anxiety (not primary, but secondary to the disease)

Aphasia (problems with the production and/or comprehension of speech)

Arrhythmia (irregular heartbeat)

Arthralgia (joint pain)

B

Back pain

Bad breath (halitosis)

Bloating of the abdomen

Blurred vision

Body odour (BO)

Bradycardia (a condition where the heart rate is slower than the accepted normal lowest rate, i.e. less than 60 beats a minute)

Brain fog (muzziness) (patients' ability to think properly about anything is usually disturbed)

Breathlessness (dyspnoea or dyspnea)

Bruising

Bruit (the name for an audible sound associated with turbulent blood flow)

Bulging eyes (exophthalmos, also known as proptosis)

C

Candidiasis (thrush or other yeast and fungal infections)

Chemical sensitivity

Clumsiness

Cognitive dysfunction

Cold hands and feet

Cold sores

Constipation

Cough

Craving for certain foods

D

Dark patches around the eyes (periorbital dark circles)

Dehydration

Depression (not primary but secondary to the disease)

Diarrhoea

Dizziness (vertigo)

Drowsiness

Dry eyes

Dry mouth

Dry skin

Dysmenorrhoea (irregular periods)

Dysphasia (aphasia)

Dyspnoea (breathlessness)

E

Earache

Electro-sensitivity (also known as electromagnetic hypersensitivity (EHS))

Endometriosis and polycystic ovary syndrome (PCOS) commonly occur together with ME/CFS and FMS and can both cause secondary dysmenorrhoea

Erectile dysfunction

F

Fainting (syncope)

Fever

Floaters (spots in your vision which appear as black or grey specks, strings or cobweb)

Forgetfulness

G

Gastroparesis (delayed gastric emptying – this is due to autonomic disturbance in ME/ CFS and FMS causing a premature full feeling while eating, nausea, gastric reflux and occasional vomiting)

Gum sores/ulcers

H

Hair loss

Hallucinations

Headache

Hearing problems

Heartburn

Hives (also known as urticaria or nettle rash)

Hyperacusis (sensitivity to loud noise)

Hyperosmia (sensitivity to smell)

Hypertension (high blood pressure)

Hyperventilation

Hypotension (low blood pressure)

I

Irritable bladder (also known as overactive bladder)

Irritable bowel (one of the most common symptoms of ME/CFS and FMS. Many patients are actually diagnosed with irritable bowel syndrome (IBS))

Itchiness (pruritus)

J

Joint pain (arthralgia)

L

Light-headedness

M

Mastalgia (breast pain)

Mastitis (inflammation in the breast)

Memory problems

Migraine

Mood swings

Myalgia (muscle pain)

N

Nausea

Neuralgia (nerve pain)

Nipple discharge (galactorrhoea)

Numbness

Nosebleeds

O

Obesity

Orthostatic intolerance (dizziness and fainting)

Overstimulation (sensory overload)

P

Pain

Palpitations (noticeable rapid, strong, or irregular heartbeats)

Perspiration problems (increased sweating, known as 'hyperhidrosis', or reduced perspiration (hypohidrosis) and, in extreme cases, anhidrosis when there is an inability to sweat at all)

Photophobia (over-sensitivity to light)

Pins-and-needles/tingling in the skin (paraesthesia)

Post-exertional malaise (PEM) (the main symptom of ME/CFS and also a major feature of FMS)

The Perrin Technique

Post-nasal drip (the constant accumulation at the back of the throat of mucus from the sinuses is caused by the inflamed mucous membranes of the nasal cavity (rhinitis))

POTS (postural orthostatic tachycardia syndrome)

Pre-menstrual syndrome (PMS)

Pressure behind the eyes and nose

R

Rosacea (an inflammatory chronic skin condition seen in ME/CFS and FMS leading to redness and raised spots)

S

Sensory overload

Sleep disturbance

Skin rashes and spots

Sore throat

Swollen glands/lymph nodes

T

Tachycardia (many patients with either ME/CFS or FMS have a rapid heartbeat of over 100 beats per minute

Temperature dysregulation (thermoregulatory disorders)

Tinnitus (continuous buzzing or ringing in the ears as well as other associated symptoms)

Toothache (often with increased sensitivity in teeth)

Temporomandibular joint (TMJ) dysfunction (jaw joint problems)

Trembling/twitching (fasciculation)

Appendix 1

U

Unrefreshing sleep

V

Vertigo (dizziness)

Vivid dreams

Voice loss (dysphonia)

Vomiting

W

Weight gain/loss

Is fibromyalgia syndrome (FMS) a different disease to ME/CFS?

Yes and no. Although there is some argument about this, I look at both of them within the same spectrum of disease, with ME/CFS producing post-exertion malaise as the principal complaint and FMS's main symptom being widespread severe pain throughout the body. It is also very important to realise that post-exertion malaise is not the same as post-exercise malaise. Often patients can exercise a little without suffering the consequences. It is exertion that precipitates the many symptoms of ME/CFS – in other words, doing more than the patient feels happy doing or capable of, and it doesn't have to be physical exertion. Mental, emotional or immunological exertion can trigger a worsening of symptoms.

I have seen some patients who were often very fit before they were ill with ME/CFS or FMS who feel much better exercising, but when they have a cold or are under emotional or mental stress they crash and may spend the next few weeks bed-ridden following perhaps an innocuous virus or extra stress at work. The reason for the different clinical presentations of FMS and ME/CFS is that the toxins in FMS predominantly affect the nuclei of the brain that control pain. This is why widespread pain is the most prominent feature in FMS rather than in ME/

CFS where the toxins mainly affect areas of the brain responsible for coping with change and preventing many other physical, emotional and cognitive problems. However, FMS and ME/CFS share the same common physical findings that we in clinic use as an aid to the diagnosis of both disorders.

As explained in detail in *The Perrin Technique 2nd Edition* symptoms of FMS are very similar to those of ME/CFS and this is why I believe they are on the same spectrum of the disease process, with FMS being diagnosed when there is widespread severe pain in all parts of the body, not just aching muscles or minor discomfort. For years, FMS was considered a rheumatologic disorder; however, the immune system has been shown to be important in the pathological process of this disease. There is much evidence to show that FMS, like ME/CFS, also arises from disturbed connections between the central autonomic nervous system, the hormonal system and the immune system.

Who suffers from these diseases?

ME/CFS and FMS can affect all ages and all ethnic groups and social backgrounds and affect men as well as women. I have recently seen a boy who has suffered the symptoms from birth, though this is extremely rare. The youngest patient with ME/ CFS I have actually treated was five years old and the oldest, 85. However, many more women suffer from ME/CFS and FMS than men. This is because:

1. Women's hormone systems are so much more complex than men's and those hormonal changes affect the hypothalamus which is the central controller of hormones in the brain and is affected by toxins in ME/CFS and FMS.
2. Levels of the cytokine leptin, which is a hormone affecting satiety and hunger and appetite or loss of it, and is found more in females, have been shown to be directly linked with the symptom severity of ME/CFS.
3. There is much more lymphatic tissue in the female breast and thus there is much more potential for congestion of the tissue in the chest, creating more toxic build-up, irritating more of the sympathetic nerves in this important area.

Appendix 1

It is interesting that at the time of writing the last stages of *The Perrin Technique 2nd Edition* in August 2020, we were starting to see in clinic a rising number of new patients with post-Covid-19 syndrome also known as 'long Covid' and that most of these post-Covid-19 patients were women. This seems to be puzzling as it has been reported worldwide that men suffer worse symptoms with Covid-19 than women and more deaths in men have been recorded due to the illness. The solution to this conundrum is the same as the reason why women develop ME/CFS and FMS much more than men as explained above.

What does the Perrin Technique treatment involve?

As described in more detail in Chapter 1, the Perrin Technique stimulates the motion of fluid around the brain and spinal cord via cranial techniques. In normal circumstances this fluid carries toxins away from the brain and spinal cord to areas of the body where they can be processed and disposed of. Treatment to the spine, as well as the exercises described in Chapter 5, further aids drainage of these toxins out of the cerebrospinal fluid. A specific lymphatic drainage technique and massage of the soft tissues in the head, neck, back and chest direct all the poisons out of the lymphatic system and into the blood, and eventually to the liver where they are broken down and readily detoxified. Some of the drainage travels out of the body via the bowels and genitourinary tract or through the skin.

Eventually, with poisons no longer affecting the central nervous system, the brain starts to work better, gradually stimulating improved lymphatic drainage. Thus, the body starts to function correctly, and, providing patients do not overstrain themselves as the nervous system is recovering, their symptoms should gradually improve.

'The rule of the artery reigns supreme.' This tenet was formulated by the founder of osteopathy, Dr Andrew Taylor Still, who stated that illness is mainly due to stagnation of body fluids and that if you can stimulate blood flow and other fluid motion, including cerebrospinal fluid and lymphatic drainage, the body will recover.

My method of treating ME/CFS, using the principle above, is analogous to mending a blocked main drain in your home. By increasing pressure into the main drain, one pumps out the blockage and reverses any backflow.

It is obviously more complex in the body, and by cranial treatment, articulation of the spine and specific manual lymphatic drainage massage techniques, one stimulates the movement of cerebrospinal fluid from the brain and the spine to the lymphatics. This increases pressure in the correct direction and thus improves the central drainage of lymph fluid from the lymphatic ducts into the blood.

What responses to treatment should I expect?

As noted in Chapter 5, one proof that the Perrin Technique is not a placebo is the fact that most patients feel somewhat worse at the beginning of the treatment. Placebo treatments do not generally make you feel worse. The reason for this initial exacerbation in symptoms is because, for the first time, the toxins embedded – for years, possibly – in the central nervous system are being released into the rest of the body.

The most common symptoms in the early stages of treatment include nausea, headaches, general pain and the appearance of spots, boils and other skin problems. However, one should always remember the old adage 'Better out than in'!

The worse the patient is in the early stage of treatment, the better the overall prognosis is usually likely to be. The main aspect to focus upon is the change that occurs with the treatment. If change has not occurred in any way in the first 12 weeks, it does not mean that the patient has no hope of recovery, but it might be a much slower process than they had envisaged. It may also mean that they have to seek an alternative/additional therapy on top of this technique in their search for a remedy. This might, for example, be medication for a chronic infection. Some fortunate patients do improve immediately, so it is not necessarily the case that a ME/CFS patient's condition worsens before improvement.

How quickly will I recover?

Every patient is different, and some recover much more quickly than others. The majority of patients improve significantly in the first year. Some mild cases can be resolved in a few months and the very severe bed-ridden patients may take years to achieve a much better quality of life, but my methods have helped some patients who had virtually given up but now are on the road to recovery (see Jade's story, page 3), with many leading a completely normal life after the treatment programme (see Table 5.3, The outlook in Chapter 5). In addition to the three case histories in this handbook, there are stories of recovery in *The Perrin Technique 2nd Edition*.

Once the patient has noticed a reduction in their symptoms, they can begin the uphill battle to improve health and stamina. One has first to convalesce, which for those younger readers who have never heard of the word, means to rest in order to get better after an illness. Convalescence is no longer a fashionable concept. People having some operations nowadays tend to be discharged from hospital within a day and may be at work within the week. Convalescent rest, however, is a must during the recovery process from ME/CFS and FMS.

In order to turn the remission period in ME/CFS and FMS into a permanent state of good health, as well as convalescence, one has to keep to the 'half rule' until one has been symptom-free for at least six months that is, doing only half of what one feels capable of doing safely. As I tell my patients, 'Remember that half of more is still more.' In other words, as one recovers and can do more before fatigue and other symptoms begin, one should only gradually increase activity, while still taking care to avoid too much exertion.

How often should I receive the Perrin Technique treatment?

At the beginning of treatment, the patient is usually treated by a licensed Perrin Technique practitioner once a week. As the symptom picture improves, there should be a gradual increase in the period between consultations. A patient with moderate symptoms with a score of 5/10 on my scale usually adheres to the following treatment schedule.

Treatment schedule

Weeks 1–12:   weekly
Weeks 13–24:   every 2 weeks
Weeks 25–36:   every 3 weeks
Weeks 37–52:   every 4 weeks
Months 12–18:   every 3 months
Month 24:   final check-up (if symptom-free for six months, patient is discharged).

However, the lower the score at the beginning, the longer it takes before recovery starts and so it may be over six months before the practitioner spaces out the weekly sessions in patients who initially score 3/10, which represents 30% of what one would call good health.

What are the dos and don'ts for patients with ME/CFS and FMS?

The answer to this question is difficult as every patient has a different presentation and what is good for one is often bad for another. However, the best way of giving a constructive response is to go through an ideal 24 hours in the life of a patient and what I have found is best advice for most.

Waking up

Let us start with getting up in the morning. It should be morning, not after midday. This is very important, as getting into a reasonably normal sleep pattern is essential. One should aim at getting up every day, and even in severe cases one should try to wake up at the same time, preferably in the morning.

The sleep-awake cycle is controlled by the hypothalamus, with the pineal gland in the brain which produces the hormone melatonin stimulated by the dark and suppressed by how much light passes through the eyes, which is why some people refer to the pineal gland as the 'third eye'. Dark and light stimulate the production of melatonin and serotonin respectively. The melatonin/serotonin balance is crucial in maintaining a good diurnal rhythm and helping us stay awake during the day and sleep at night.

In the winter the darker days aggravate the rhythm and some people suffer a drop in serotonin and become more depressed, leading to what is known as SAD (seasonal affective disorder). Also, many ME/CFS and FMS patients sleep much worse in the summer as they have too little melatonin and too much in the winter. To help the balance in winter, a SAD light which mimics daylight hours does often help. So, if you have this problem, a SAD light is important first thing in the morning at dawn for an hour, and another hour later on in the evening at twilight/dusk is also recommended.

Getting out of bed

If this is possible (and unfortunately I have seen many patients who are unable to lift their heads off a pillow, never mind get out of bed), always alight from the bed in stages; never jump up as the control over blood pressure is often disturbed and experiencing dizziness when getting out of bed is common. So, before sitting up make sure you are lying on your side and slowly swing your legs over the edge of the bed and gradually sit up at the side of your bed where you should remain for a minute or so before slowly standing up. If you suffer from POTS (postural orthostatic tachycardia syndrome – see *The Perrin Technique 2nd Edition*, Chapter 5, page 172) you should stay seated for at least three minutes before trying to stand up.

Shower in the morning

This should never be too hot or too cold as the hypothalamus is the thermostat of the body and too extreme temperatures will stress an already overloaded part of the brain. Make sure any soaps, shampoos and shower-gels are not too perfumed. It is worth buying the least allergenic products recommended by your local pharmacist even if they are more expensive.

Try to avoid hot baths at any time. They are worse than showers as besides overheating the body, the muscles will relax while the spine is in an unhealthy position unless you are able to float in the bath. It always amazes me as an osteopath how many people take a hot bath when they have lower back pain. Sitting in the bath places extra strain on the lower back and can aggravate any postural problem. With ME/CFS and FMS it is double trouble as the heat and the postural strain together exacerbate any inflammatory changes in the spine, which creates more toxicity within the central nervous system.

Comfortably cool baths that you can lie in are healthier for ME/CFS and FMS patients and sometimes relieve many of the symptoms, but if the water is too cold it will aggravate the condition by increasing tone in already tightened muscles. If you are going to try cool baths, make sure that when you are lying there you are not shivering and that you are comfortable. I recommend about 10 minutes at a time.

Showers are usually better for ME/CFS but if the patient feels dizzy or weak standing and does not have a bath then they should use a shower chair. If a patient constantly feels faint or actually faints in a hot shower and the heart rate frequently races, then again suspect possible POTS.

Having frequent short cold showers of around 16–23°C may also be of benefit to some ME/CFS and FMS patients. As with cool baths, moderately cold showers have been shown to reduce pain by stimulating the production of endorphins which reduce pain without causing any harm.

Cool showers and baths have been shown to stimulate the locus coeruleus in the brain stem which forms a major axis, together with the hypothalamus, in the control mechanism of the neuro-lymphatic drainage system. In health this axis switches off during the night in deep restorative delta-wave sleep. It has been shown that in ME/CFS, delta-waves are produced in the brain throughout the day

Appendix 1

with the axis switching off at the wrong time leading to the patient feeling sick and exhausted as the toxins drain out of the brain. To reverse this problem, we need to stimulate the locus coeruleus during the day. So brief, comfortably cool hydrotherapy in the morning will greatly help some patients.

Exposure to cold typically causes activation of the sympathetic nervous system (SNS) which can cause problems with ME/CFS and FMS since the sympathetic nerves are usually overloaded. However, small amounts of stressful or harmful agents can sometimes be beneficial. This phenomenon is known as hormesis. Similar to the body's immune response needing to first be exposed to an infectious agent before it builds an immunity, as seen in vaccination, it is believed by some that exposure to cold can temporarily reverse autonomic dysfunction and therefore improve symptoms.

If your symptoms are improving with the manual therapy in this book but you wish to boost your energy, try the hydrotherapy once in the morning for just a few minutes, either lying in a cool bath or having bursts of a cold shower for a few seconds at a time over a couple of minutes. If it brings any relief, continue each morning as long as you always feel well afterwards. If it worsens your condition in any way, then immediately stop as it isn't for you. Remember that every ME/CFS and FMS patient is different, and unfortunately people respond differently to any stimulus.

On that note, there is a completely different form of hydrotherapy developed in Japan that has been shown to relieve mental fatigue. This is known as 'mild stream bathing' which involves a mild stream of warm water continuously passing from the sole to the calf, thigh, waist and back, providing a massage function. This form of therapy would stimulate lymphatic drainage, working against any backflow, so it may help ME/CFS and FMS as long as the water isn't too hot. It should only be attempted in the later stages of treatment as full body massage could easily overload the drainage of toxins and be too much for your body to cope with when embarking on the Perrin Technique.

Getting dressed

Loose clothes that are easy to slip on and off are recommended as clothing that is too tight may restrict circulation of blood and lymph and lots of buttons etc can place strain on the hands that do get fatigued and sometimes become very painful, especially in FMS. For women, tight bras are a definite no-no, especially tight underwired bras, which do place extra pressure on the breast lymphatics. Sports bras tend to be better, but the main issue is finding a properly fitted bra; bra-fitting services should be used and are available at good quality shops around the world.

Deodorants, antiperspirants and cosmetics

Most should be avoided as much as possible, especially heavily perfumed products as they usually contain high levels of petrochemicals and other neurotoxins. There are safer products that are less toxic, but one has to shop around. In the same vein, many of my patients relax by lighting scented candles at home. Unfortunately, aromatic candles are nearly all highly toxic, with the wax usually having a high petrochemical content and the wicks usually containing heavy metals. If you enjoy candles to relax, please try and use beeswax ones with natural, non-metallic wicks.

Mealtimes

Diets are discussed at length in Chapter 5 of *The Perrin Technique 2nd Edition*, but the basic advice I give is not to eat anything in excess and generally 'Variety is the spice of life'. Eating a large variety of foods generally places less strain on a particular part of the gastrointestinal system, which is often disturbed in ME/CFS and FMS patients, with many having irritable bowel syndrome and gut dysbiosis.

Dietary intake of sugar should be low as it stimulates the production of yeast. Patients with ME/CFS and FMS should eat less casein (found in milk-based products), less gluten, as well as less yeast, as these are all composed of large molecules and therefore require the lymphatics to drain the excess away from the gut.

Small meals eaten regularly are best and I often advise patients to divide each meal into two, eating frequently but less at a time. Adults should drink around

Appendix 1

2 litres of water a day and/or healthy drinks such as herbal non-caffeinated teas. Patients should reduce the intake of caffeinated coffee and tea as caffeine can over-stimulate the nervous system. Alcohol should be avoided at all costs as, besides it obviously placing extra strain on the liver, it has been shown that patients with ME/CFS and FMS have overactive receptors in the brain that are stimulated by NMDA, the neurochemical activated by alcohol intake. Most of my patients do not find this advice difficult to follow as they feel worse after a little sip and almost drunk following the smallest amount of alcohol.

Chillax (chill and relax)

During the day and especially at night the patient has to learn how to relax and possibly meditate. A new word has been coined that embodies both relaxing and remaining chilled and calm: 'Chillax'. There are plenty of different strategies mentioned in Chapter 5 of *The Perrin Technique 2nd Edition* to do this, including mindfulness.

Bedtime

Difficulty falling asleep and staying asleep, known as insomnia, and hypersomnia, when the patient sleeps too much, and other sleep disturbances, are very common symptoms of ME/CFS and FMS. Leading sleep experts including Dr Jason Ellis, who is a Professor of Sleep Science and Director of the Northumbria Sleep Research Laboratory in the UK, advocate cognitive behavioural therapy for insomnia, often called CBT-I.

CBT-I is an approved method for treating insomnia aimed at changing sleep habits and includes regular, often weekly, visits to a clinician and completing a sleep diary to work out the best way of tackling the specific disorder.

Sleep clinics around the world offer many ways of analysing the sleep problem and for those patients with severe sleep disorders a polysomnography test is essential. Also known as a sleep study test, polysomnography records your brain waves, the oxygen level in your blood, heart rate and breathing, as well as eye and leg movements.

Exercises to help you to fall asleep should be attempted, such as counting backwards from a thousand ... in sevens – i.e. 1000, 993, 986, 979 etc. It isn't easy and that is the main point. By taking your mind off everything else your brain will be calmer and you will gently fall asleep. At the same time it can also help if you think 'I am not going to sleep ... I am not going to sleep' and repeat this over and over again in your mind while counting down from 1000 in 7s.

It is best to have a set bedtime and stick to it as closely as possible. Use blackout curtains and switch off all lights in the room. It's best to take all the electronic gadgets away from the bed. Avoid tea, coffee and any other drinks with caffeine before bed.

Sometimes having a small meal an hour before bed helps. As one knows after a heavy meal during the day, one often feels very drowsy. This is because hormones released after eating can also stimulate the sleep centres. These hormones are controlled by the hypothalamus which is, as we have seen, the main part of the brain disturbed in ME/ CFS and FMS. Eating food can calm the hypothalamus and help induce sleep.

The best position for sleep is lying on one's side, which places minimal strain on to the spine. It has also been shown that neuro-lymphatic drainage occurs more when lying on one's side (no particular side, just the one you feel more comfortable on).

Some patients may develop sleep apnoea, which is when one stops breathing during one's sleep for short periods. This obviously can be dangerous ... we need to breathe; so contact your GP if you think you have this problem. You may need an aid to support breathing at night called a continuous positive airway pressure machine (CPAP), which is the most effective treatment if you have moderate to severe sleep apnoea.

Sleeping pills and low-dose tricyclic antidepressants, such as 10 mg amitriptyline, are prescribed by GPs to be taken an hour before bed. Some patients taking amitriptyline report feeling very drowsy the next morning, so if you have a problem inform your GP. As mentioned in the beginning of this section, the hormone melatonin is important for sleep so sometimes this is prescribed by physicians around the world to help ME/CFS patients sleep, but the SAD light (page 105) may be the best help.

How much exercise and activity can I do?

Post-*exertion* malaise (PEM) is the most common symptom in ME/CFS … not, as I have said on many occasions throughout this book, post-*exercise* malaise. Any activity that does not over-exert you will be okay and activity is actively encouraged if possible, as long as it does not exhaust you. PEM may not be immediate; the malaise may kick in up to three days following exertion, so beware of this problem.

It is best to avoid all exertive exercise and sport until you are virtually symptom free and then you can revitalise your deconditioned body by gradually increasing your activity. The dreaded graded exercise therapy (GET) helps only ME/CFS and FMS patients who are fortunate enough to have recovered from most of their symptoms but, due to the forced reduction of activity over a protracted period, are deconditioned. Even when their concentration returns and when feeling much more energetic, they still often remain basically unfit and one of the best ways of reconditioning the body is by gradually increasing physical activity.

Rehabilitation and reconditioning patients' weakened bodies has to be done safely. The best rehabilitative activity for the recovering ME/CFS and FMS patient is a swimming stroke known as adapted back sculling (see Figure 34), which is done lying on the back and gently wafting the arms along just beneath the water surface, slowly propelling you backwards; however, with this rehabilitative exercise you should slowly move your legs up and down as well.

Avoid breaststroke as this is just wrong on so many levels. When I was specialising in sports injuries the top-level swimmers that I saw most were the breast-stroke swimmers. This is the most common stroke among casual swimmers but places unnatural strain on the neck, shoulders, spine, pelvis, hips and knees … besides that, it's okay.

The Perrin Technique

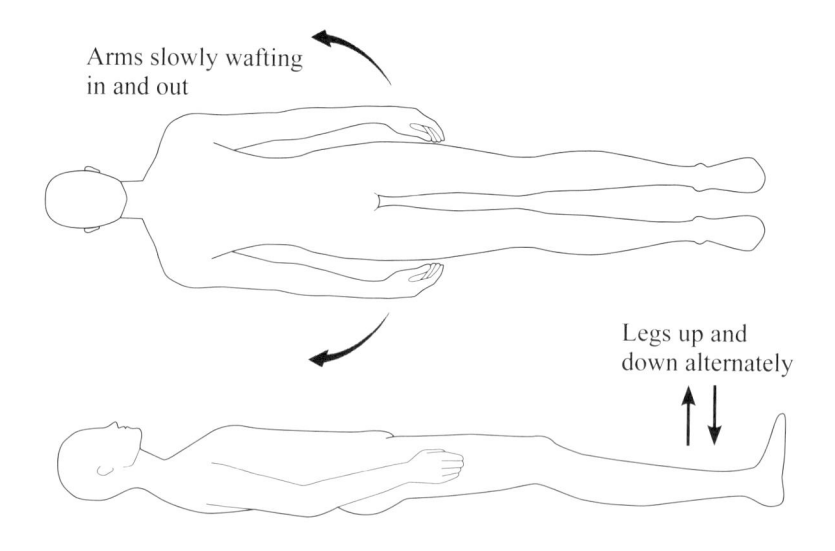

Fig. 34 Adapted back sculling technique

As you are able to do more, then you can introduce backstroke and front crawl but try not to break any speed and distance records. One of my patients once threw caution to the wind and as soon as she felt able to swim a few lengths she decided to swim a couple of kilometres and spent the next few months in bed, recovering. Swimming in a saltwater pool, if one is available, or the sea if it is not too cold, is preferable to a chlorinated pool due to the toxic effects of the chlorine.

As the symptoms continue to improve, both the patient and the practitioner will be greatly encouraged. By steadily improving the mobility of the spine, and by relaxing all the irritated surrounding tissues, the function of the sympathetic nervous system should finally be restored to full working order. The patient once again enjoys health, vigour and a good quality of life and hopefully can go back to a more active lifestyle exercising in gyms and playing sports.

However, ... never forget my golden rule for any activity – what I call the 'half rule', i.e. only do 50% of what you feel capable of. This rule applies to activity, including walking, talking, reading, writing and watching television. However,

Appendix 1

when it comes to aerobic exercise such as running and swimming, the patient has to be absolutely sure that they will not go over the half rule or risk a major relapse.

As I always say to my patients, and have said above: 'Half of more is still more.' In other words, when increasing exercise, doing a little at a time, if you are well within your safe boundaries, will still increase your stamina and general fitness, with no risk.

The half rule is so difficult to adhere to because, once on the mend, it is as though the patient's prison door has been unlocked for the first time in maybe years and yet they are only allowed to walk around the courtyard and then go back into their cell. However, if one were to run out of the prison gates too quickly, the guns and dogs of ME/CFS and FMS would be there ready to stop the fleeing prisoner in their tracks. Much better to walk calmly out through the gates at a very gentle pace and then stop and return for a while and then go a bit further the next time, continually returning to the safety of the cell for a while, until one can slowly but surely leave the ME/CFS or FMS prison without alerting the sympathetic nervous system's 'prison guards' that one has escaped their clutches.

Patients who are eager to resume some form of aerobic exercise and can't swim, or live too far from a swimming pool or suitable beach, or remain sensitive to chlorine, should begin by gentle walks up and down the street and gradually increase the distance. Walking should be on the flat at the beginning of rehabilitation and, if possible, while wearing a pedometer, which is a device that counts each step a person takes by detecting movement of the arms or hips; this is a very useful tool to monitor the gentle progress that you should be aiming for.

A pedometer can simply be downloaded as an app for your phone or you can buy a simple device in most sports supply shops. Gradually increase the activity, keeping to walking and not jogging: shifting all one's weight onto first one side and then the other places too much strain on the spine whereas walking avoids this jarring effect.

Cycling should only be done on the flat. As with walking, avoid hills to begin with as this may over-exert your back and leg muscles. A basic exercise bike with a little resistance is also a good form of rehabilitation.

REMEMBER: graded activity does not help ME/CFS and FMS patients recover but helps re-condition the recovered patient!

What hobbies can I do safely?

Hobbies and pastimes are very important for patients' sense of purpose and sanity, especially if housebound. They can also be a crucial part of rehabilitation, reintroducing physical and mental activity to a life that has just been about existing from day to day. If the hobby involves arts and crafts, the patient may be suffering neurotoxicity from the paint, paint thinners and solvents they use. These and many other hobbies involving toxins should be kept to a minimum for obvious reasons. Patients should wear a mask if there is any danger of exposure to poisonous fumes.

Playing a musical instrument is a favourite among some patients as they increase their abilities. This is highly recommended, but again try to space out the sessions whatever instrument you enjoy playing, and when playing the piano, to begin with, use a supportive chair rather than a standard piano stool as sitting with no back support will place extra strain on your spine.

If recovering patients take to gardening, they have to be careful not to expose themselves to organophosphates, such as pesticides and herbicides. Also, patients should invest in tools with long handles that reduce the need to stretch and bend. Be careful when carrying out repetitive actions to prevent overstraining weakened muscles.

Is technology safe to use?

People always think watching TV is a very passive activity and cannot overload the nervous system. They couldn't be more wrong. TV images create a hive of neuronal activity in the brain as one has to digest what is going on in each scene of a play, film or even a gameshow or the news. Screens also send out 'blue light', which has been shown to stimulate alpha-waves, as mentioned in Chapter 1 (page 12). During the morning blue light is beneficial as it boosts mood, reaction times and concentration, but in the evening, and especially just before bed, it reduces good restorative sleep, so the advice to all patients is: do not watch TV for at least an hour before bed. A recent survey by a leading phone manufacturer found that almost nine out of 10 18–34-year-olds have trouble sleeping because they use their smartphones at bedtime. Technology firms have acknowledged the problem, with some major mobile tech providers introducing special settings that reduce blue light. Special yellow or orange tinted glasses can be used to filter out the harmful blue light.

Blue-light-filter glasses or blue-light-filter apps should definitely be used if using a computer for long periods. Many of my younger patients spend much of their day playing on computer games or looking at their phones. These screens should be set up with filters that shield the blue light as the day draws to a close. As with TV, all screens should be avoided for an hour before bed even when using the filter.

I recommend listening to relaxing music, reading or, if reading is difficult, listening to a talking book last thing at night as a good alternative.

Any screen-time should be restricted during the day as spending too long in one position can lead to postural strain on the spine and repetitive strain injuries when using game consoles or texting. Muscles are much more susceptible to damage from constant repetitive trauma, especially in FMS. Hands-free options and non-metal cases on phones should be used to reduce radio frequency exposure.

When can I return to work/education?

If you have been off sick from work for a protracted amount of time, as you improve and are well enough to start work, you should never consider just returning to work full-time as soon as you feel better. You need to gradually increase hours in a phased return-to-work programme, as shown in Table 11.1 (page 350) in *The Perrin Technique 2nd Edition*. The phased return schedule depends on many factors and differs from patient to patient.

The rule of thumb is that you should listen to your body and symptoms. In other words, if you are struggling mid-way through the phased return programme and find four hours a day too much, you can go back a week or two in the schedule.

A similar situation occurs when a young patient is out of full-time or part-time education due to ME/CFS and FMS. Pressure to place the young person back into school is often compounded by social services becoming involved. Parents continue to be suspected of making their child worse than they actually are. Conditions like 'Munchausen's disease by proxy' and 'fictitious illness syndrome' have been mentioned by the authorities, at times accusing patients' parents of making their children feel ill without any real physical cause of the disease.

Once the young person begins to improve, they can return to school, maybe just at break-time to begin with, so that there is some social interaction with their peer group. Little by little, add an extra class into the phased return schedule, and as long as the young person feels that they are not getting too tired, they should continue to build up their attendance.

University courses often present a problem as one cannot usually attend full-time degrees in a part-time capacity unless one joins a part-time course. This should sometimes be considered if the illness is too severe to continue. Another alternative is for severe patients to defer their university place for a time and hopefully they will be able to return to their studies once recovered. This has been the case with many of my student patients and most go on to receive a much better degree than if they had tried to struggle through. I am so proud of many of my patients who defer their university course and end up with excellent final exam results, going on to flourishing careers.

Are there any dos and don'ts on commuting?

Travelling to and from work and school should always be factored into any phased return. Any travelling that places the patient under too much strain should be avoided. Going by train for long distances is usually better than driving as sitting for long periods can easily harm the spine. On the train the patient can get up and walk around a little as well as have a rest without the extra stress of traffic jams.

If I am improving can I go on holiday?

When you are well enough to take a vacation, it shouldn't first be a long-haul flight to a country that is very hot. Patients need to shelter from too much sun. Symptoms of both ME/CFS and FMS are exacerbated by jet lag, excessive temperatures and sunburn.

Often it's not the holiday that harms the patient, and a beach with fresh air and some sun and shelter, with the occasional dip into the sea, is often the best place to be. The problem lies in getting there and airports with their queues, and the long distances to the gate can be very damaging to the patient.

So, when flying I always advise patients who haven't yet recovered to order wheelchair support at airports. However much the patient may dislike the public display of their illness, they never regret following this advice since most airport staff look after wheelchair passengers and their families really well and take all the stress out of the airport experience.

If you have to go on a long-haul flight that may induce jet lag, ask your doctor or pharmacist about melatonin to take after the long flight, especially one that is travelling eastwards, such as from the USA to Europe. Melatonin helps to regulate the body's circadian rhythm and helps some patients' sleep problems. It is prescribed off-label for jet lag in many countries, but it is best to ask your doctor's advice before taking it.

When on holiday in a hot climate, make sure you keep in the shade as much as possible and use the highest-rated sunblock. Sunburn will aggravate the pain in FMS and ME/CFS so you need to avoid direct sun when possible. Try to avoid overheating and going to winter resorts that are too cold, as both will strain your hypothalamus, which is the body's thermostat, as discussed earlier. The best option is to go on vacation where the weather isn't too extreme.

Is it safe to get pregnant with ME/CFS or FMS?

There are two viewpoints concerning pregnancy and ME/CFS. Some experts believe that pregnancy is a time when a better balance is achieved within the woman's body and it can help reduce the symptoms of ME/CFS. However, this is unpredictable. Some healthy women blossom when pregnant; if the ME/CFS patient is lucky enough to be that type, her symptoms will probably reduce during pregnancy. However, if the mother-to-be is one of those who generally have a difficult pregnancy, her ME/CFS symptoms may worsen for most of the nine months as her hormone levels fluctuate, producing more nausea and fatigue.

ME/CFS and especially FMS present a problem for the actual delivery of the baby as the natural pain in childbirth will be exacerbated and aggravate the widespread pain due to the illness. Gas and air or hypnosis should be considered before opting for any other forms of anaesthetic for the birth itself.

From a positional point of view, the best position for patients giving birth is the left lateral position, which is still commonly used and reduces strain on the spine compared with any other position.

If local or general anaesthetics are used in the labour, then one should check that they are safe and are non-adrenaline (epinephrine) based.

If there is a choice between having a spinal block or electing to have a Caesarean section, I would opt for the latter as injecting an anaesthetic directly into the spine is definitely not recommended for patients with ME/CFS and FMS.

A study published in 2004 showed that ME/CFS symptoms improve in about one third of pregnant ME/CFS patients, usually after the first trimester, and are unchanged in about one third and worsen in about one third, with worsening symptoms in their second and later pregnancies. Any supplements taken for ME/CFS should be confirmed by your doctor as safe to take during pregnancy.

It's not just the pregnancy; it's the baby afterwards that obviously places more strain on the mother, and this is more of a problem. I would usually advise a patient to wait

Appendix 1

until they are well on the mend before they consider pregnancy. A survey found that 21% of a group of ME/CFS patients decided not to have a child because they thought that their debility would interfere with their ability to raise their child.

Breastfeeding carries the risk of toxins being transferred from mother to baby, so the best advice regarding this factor is for the mother to have as much detox treatment as possible before she plans on getting pregnant.

There is also the genetic factor to consider. There is a 15% chance of ME/CFS being familial (running in families). However, I would never advise patients not to have children because they don't want the risk of them also getting the disease. I do believe ME/CFS is preventable, with the physical signs (see page 36) appearing before the symptoms, so if a patient is worried about his/her child developing the illness, the child can be assessed for the five physical signs and if there is a problem they can be treated with the manual techniques before any symptoms arise. The physical signs will reduce quickly, and the child should remain healthy.

If I require surgery, what precautions are needed?

You may have other problems that require an operation. If surgery is not essential, I would advise a delay as long as possible until you have improved with my treatment. However, occasionally surgery is crucial and needs to be done as soon as possible. In these cases, the advice I give to patients about general anaesthetics is that the anaesthetist should be aware of the illness and to follow the advice of one of the leading experts in this field, American physician and ME/CFS specialist Dr Charles Lapp.

Some patients have low magnesium and potassium levels so Dr Lapp recommends pre-operative tests for serum magnesium and potassium should be done as low levels can affect the heart under anaesthesia.

Many ME/CFS and FMS patients, especially the very severe, housebound patients, have a problem with their hypothalamic-pituitary-adrenal axis affecting their adrenal glands. Therefore, Dr Lapp also advises that cortisol levels should be tested before any operation, as low levels could place the patient at risk, so supplements may be required before surgery can commence.

All supplements should be discussed with the anaesthetist to check that they will be safe to take and that they will not interfere with the surgery or the anaesthetic. If possible, it is usually sensible to avoid most supplements for two weeks before surgery, especially garlic, ginseng and *Gingko biloba*, which increase bleeding.

Most of my patients have managed to recover quite quickly post-surgery, as long as they have taken things very easy and convalesced after their ordeal. The days of convalescent homes are long gone but, when patients return home from hospital, they should be very careful to pace their activity to avoid a relapse of their symptoms.

How important are environmental factors?

All of us are exposed to a number of pollutants in our everyday lives. ME/CFS sufferers need to minimise as far as possible their exposure to these toxins (see Chapter 3).

Sometimes it is not patients themselves who are directly exposed to a pollutant or environmental toxin. It can often be a family member who may be an engineer, a hairdresser or a car-paint sprayer. Many patients have had a possible neuro-lymphatic drainage problem since birth and have been harmed by living in a household where one or both parents have jobs that bring them into increased contact with toxins. The parents come home and may hug their baby and wash their clothes in the same machine as their child's clothes. This cross-contamination over the years can lead to the gradual build-up of neurotoxins in the brain and spinal cord, with the child eventually having sufficient exposure to trigger the onset of ME/CFS or FMS. Sometimes the onset of illness is many years later when the patient is an adult. Medicines for babies and children are given in minimal dosages since the young are much more susceptible to the effects of toxins, illustrating the fact that in the young toxic exposure does not have to be great to inflict harm.

Appendix 1

When visiting the dentist, avoid having mercury amalgam dental fillings. When going to have your hair done at the hair salon, the use of chemicals in your hair should be limited, especially since some have been shown to harm the actual hairdresser. Remember that the scalp is very close to the brain and it is not advisable to massage poisons into the skin in this area. Take care to make sure that your neck is in a comfortable position, too, when your hair is being washed in a back basin.

Patients who are hairdressers themselves, or in other occupations that use large amounts of toxic materials, should take extra measures to avoid further exposure, such as wearing gloves and masks and having plenty of ventilation. This is advice that is all too familiar during the Covid-19 outbreak, but any patient working with toxins should continue to take these measures after the pandemic is over.

If you live in the countryside, take a trip away from home during crop spraying days. If your work entails exposure to harmful toxins, you may need to consider a career change.

If both spouses or a few people in the same street develop ME/CFS or FMS, then try and see if there are any sources of pollution close by that may be a cause. One case that comes to mind is a couple who both were suffering from severe symptoms of ME/CFS. They were not blood related and yet both had been ill for a few years. They had been living in the same house for 20 years with their own little herb and vegetable garden, with no factories, farms or large roads nearby and their own market garden was 100% organic. They were not living under a flight path and they both had jobs that did not involve any contact with any toxins.

It seemed a very unusual case and, with the prevalence of ME/CFS on the increase, it could have been an unfortunate coincidence that the couple both had ME/CFS from other triggers rather than environmental. However, toxic screening at a local lab showed they both had high levels of nickel and cadmium in their blood samples. On questioning I found out that when they moved into their home it was a new build and further investigation revealed that it was built on a landfill site. I enquired about what the estate was built on and it was not so surprising they were being poisoned as the house was directly on top of a demolished car battery factory! Nickel and cadmium are used in the production of rechargeable batteries and obviously there was a seepage from the factory ruins into the soil. Sadly, this husband and wife both had different previous mechanical problems that had compromised their neuro-lymphatic pathways. However, the large amount of vegetables and herbs grown in this poisoned soil, and eaten for many years by this unfortunate couple, lay behind their illness.

As I said above, candles and scented products at home should be used sparingly as they are full of petrochemicals. If you move into a new home and you have new carpets, curtains and other soft furnishings, make sure you have plenty of ventilation. When decorating, use low-odour paint and again it is best to stay out of the house when the paint is being applied, especially the gloss. Make sure any home gas appliances are not emitting harmful carbon monoxide; ensure that you have detectors fitted in your home. Also, if you live in a damp, older property have an environmental check for mould.

When using mobile phones make sure you use a hands-free option as much as possible as holding it close to the head has been shown to damage the blood–brain barrier, making the brain more vulnerable to toxins.

Can the Perrin Technique help with other conditions?

This is a tricky question to answer. The simple answer is yes. Over the years, I have had the wonderful pleasure of working alongside some amazing doctors. One is leading neurologist Dr Margareta Griesz-Brisson in Harley Street, London. She always says: 'Ray, we are treating the physiology not the pathology.' In other words, the treatment is designed to aid the restoration of a healthy neuro-lymphatic system, which physiologically will encourage the central nervous system to work better. So, many problems affecting the nervous system should be helped by the Perrin Technique.

Appendix 1

There are other diseases linked to problems affecting the lymphatic drainage of the brain. Scans in 2012 revealed visible proof of the drainage of beta amyloid proteins out of the brains of mice via the perivascular spaces into the lymphatic system. This showed how these large molecules could stagnate in diseases such as Alzheimer's, which has been linked to the accumulation of beta amyloid plaques, which destroy connections between the brain's neurones, affecting thinking, memory and behaviour.

I have treated a few patients with Alzheimer's disease and one elderly man in the early stages of the disorder received once a month treatment for four years with no deterioration in his symptoms throughout the four years. In fact, he sometimes came in for his monthly session saying he had had the best month yet, with increased energy and concentration and memory as good as ever. Sadly, he subsequently had a fall and injured his head which led to a speedy deterioration in his condition.

Another condition that I have helped many patients with over the years is Lyme disease; with this infection, the reverse flow of lymphatic drainage leads to a build-up of the bacterium *Borrelia burgdorferi* in the central nervous system. Research has also shown that problems with lymphatic drainage of the brain may also lead to some forms of clinical depression and rarer conditions such as Creutzfeldt-Jakob disease (CJD).

The neuro-lymphatic drainage pathway was shown to be affected in patients with the severe acute respiratory syndrome (SARS) caused by the coronavirus infection of 2003, with some developing a ME/CFS-like illness. The coronavirus in Covid-19 seems to be causing the same post-viral fatigue states, leading to a post-Covid-19 syndrome (long Covid), which has all the hallmarks of ME/CFS, and could very well affect the drainage in the olfactory pathway leading to loss of smell and taste, and an effect on the hypothalamus leading to high fever. In May 2020, I saw a 42-year-old man in clinic who responded very well to neuro-lymphatic treatment a month after having had severe post-Covid-19 symptoms and who was completely symptom-free two months later. We are seeing more and more post-Covid-19 patients in clinic with all the physical signs and many symptoms of ME/CFS and most will respond very quickly to the Perrin Technique if caught in the first few months after coming down with the virus.

As the lymphatic drainage of the brain is being further investigated by neuroscientists around the world, more conditions will probably be connected to the dysfunction of this important process. This will probably indicate the validity in using the techniques shown in this book to treat many other neurological diseases that, at the time of writing, have no successful treatment and continue to baffle the medical world.

Once I have recovered, can the illness recur?

As patients recover, if they overdo things, suffer from infections or have to cope with too much stress, their symptoms may return or worsen. Some patients do suffer recurrences when they have significantly improved, but few experience relapses once they have been discharged, unless they push themselves too far day after day. ME/CFS and FMS patients, once recovered, need to reassess their lifestyle and take steps to reduce the continual stress that may have been part of what led to the illness in the first place. One should be able to exert oneself when better, but knowing when to stop is important.

Patients who have been discharged should continue the dorsal rotation exercises (pages 61-63) three times a day for life. Self-massage to the chest and neck should be done once a week in the shower. An annual check-up is advisable.

Should a relapse occur, it may take a long time to reverse, but remember that, if the treatment worked the first time, it should work again and perhaps more quickly the second time. Psychologists and counsellors are invaluable in these cases. The important rule in treatment, and even more so after relapse, is to remain as positive as possible. Negative thoughts create further neurotoxicity.

To secure a permanent remission and to remain in good health, one has to focus on the task ahead by means of sensible pacing (the '50% rule'), thus achieving a slow but sure return to good health.

Following a graded exercise programme, but only when better, is a good idea, not to treat the ME/CFS or FMS itself, but to help recondition the body and to remain fit and well in the future.

Can ME/CFS and FMS be prevented?

I am one of the few practitioners who maintain that ME/CFS and FMS can be prevented. The physical signs are very real and usually are seen long before the symptoms begin. This is why in the very early stages of the disorder only a physical and postural-based examination can detect the development of these disorders before the sympathetic nervous system breaks down.

If ME/CFS or FMS is found in more than one family member, there is probably a genetic predisposition that leads to a restricted flow of toxins from the brain and spine. I have discovered when examining children, siblings or even parents of the patient that they present some or all of the five physical signs of ME/CFS and FMS (See Figure 8, page 36).

When treating pre-ME, as I call it, the signs significantly reduce, usually with only a few weeks or months of treatment. For this reason, I believe that ME/CFS is preventable if treated and managed properly in the early stages.

The advice to physicians given by the International Association of CFS/ME states that establishing a diagnosis of ME/CFS as soon as possible will usually give the patient a much greater chance of relief.

The very severe cases of patients in bed all day and night in silent, darkened rooms should never happen, as early diagnosis should then be followed up quickly with advice on pacing and the appropriate treatment. The severe cases may be as a result of the wrong treatment or bad advice being given in the early stages of the illness, with patients being instructed and sometimes coerced to increase their activity, and sometimes medicated with drugs that have severe effects on the central nervous system.

If all practitioners around the world were taught to examine patients for the early physical signs, which are evidence-based, and to carefully review the patient's history and symptoms for indications and signs of neurotoxicity, there would be far fewer severe cases. If patients were given advice to pace at the outset, together with prompt treatment to restore a healthy neuro-lymphatic system, it could help prevent ME/CFS and FMS developing in the first place, and one day make these terribly cruel illnesses a thing of the past.

Appendix 2

Common pathological and radiological tests

Around the world, most ME/CFS and FMS patients are diagnosed by exclusion, since there is no definitive diagnostic pathological test from blood or other body fluid samples that can accurately diagnose these disorders. Hopefully, by using the methods detailed in this book, clinicians will be able to reach a definite positive diagnosis, but since there are many comorbidities that can cause similar symptoms to ME/CFS and FMS one has to initially carry out many pathological tests to see the complete picture. Clinically, due to the overall disturbance in the general metabolic processes in ME/CFS and FMS patients, many of the blood tests carried out are usually in the high or low range, but the values tend to remain just within the normal boundaries.

Many of my patients when we first meet hand me the results of dozens of lab tests ordered by their doctor without really understanding what they were for. Over and above what I include here, there are many more blood, urine, stool and salivary tests plus an incredible array of scans that can now be carried out to test for all sorts of conditions that may be the cause of some of the patient's symptoms. However, this section deals with the most frequent tests that doctors usually request when they are looking for an explanation of some or many of the symptoms which present in ME/CFS.

Since there is a difference from lab to lab across the world regarding what is considered a normal healthy range I have purposely left out a reference range. Most labs include reference ranges for normal on individual test results so make sure you have the results explained to you by the lab or your own GP.

Antibody tests

- **Rheumatoid factor (RF)**: Rheumatoid factor is an antibody that is measurable in the blood that can bind to other antibodies. Up to 70–90% of patients with rheumatoid arthritis (RA) have a positive RF test. The RF test is not diagnostic. It must be interpreted in conjunction with the patient's symptoms and history, and with tests of inflammation such as ESR or CRP (see page 129). RF is also present in patients with other conditions, including other connective tissue diseases (such as systemic lupus erythematosus), some infectious diseases, liver disease and sarcoidosis. RF can also sometimes be present in healthy people who have RA in the family.

- **ANF (anti-nuclear factor) or ANA (anti-nuclear antibody)**: The ANF or ANA test is carried out to check for systemic lupus erythematosus (SLE) or other connective tissue disorders. However, a positive ANF test by itself is not proof of SLE. Another test – antibody to double stranded DNA measurement – is used to determine if the symptoms may be due to SLE.

- **Complement component 3 and 4**: Complement component is a blood test that measures the activity of a certain protein that is part of the innate immune complement system that plays a part in the development of inflammation. C3 and C4 are the most commonly measured complement components. Complement activity may be measured to determine how severe a disease is or if treatment is working.

- **Endomysial antibody**: This is a test for the autoimmune response to gluten seen in coeliac disease.

Appendix 2

Full blood count

In a full blood count, the blood sample is well mixed and placed on a rack of an analyser which is an instrument that measures different elements in the blood. The detailed analysis will examine the blood cells for the following values.

Red blood cells (the oxygen-carrying cells in blood)

- Total red blood cells: The numbers of red blood cells (RBCs) are given as an absolute number per litre.
- Haemoglobin: The amount of haemoglobin in the blood, expressed in grams per decilitre (low haemoglobin = anaemia).
- Haematocrit or packed cell volume (PCV): This is the fraction of whole blood volume that consists of red blood cells.
- Red blood cell indices or mean corpuscular volume (MCV): The average volume of the red cells, measured in femtolitres (10–15 litres). Anaemia is classified as microcytic or macrocytic based on whether this value is above or below the expected normal range.
- Mean corpuscular haemoglobin (MCH): The average amount of haemoglobin per red blood cell, measured in picograms (10-15 of a kilogram).
- Mean corpuscular haemoglobin concentration (MCHC): The average concentration of haemoglobin in the cells.
- Red blood cell distribution width (RDW): This is a measure of the variation across the RBC population.

Other blood cell counts

- **White blood cells** (the cells in the blood needed for the immune system): The total white blood cells are given as a percentage and as an absolute number per litre.
- **Platelets** (the cells in the blood needed for clotting).

- **Immune cells**: A complete blood count will include the numbers of specific immune cells, such as neutrophils, lymphocytes, monocytes, eosinophils and basophils.

Other common blood tests

- **Calcium (Ca)**: A calcium blood test is important as calcium is one of the main minerals needed for bone and muscle integrity and is also essential for proper functioning of your nerves and heart.
- **C-reactive protein (CRP)**: CRP is produced in the liver and its level in the blood will rise in response to inflammation, so it is a very accurate marker for any inflammatory state. Typically, patients with ME/CFS and FMS have a low to normal CRP; however, a higher than normal level can occur but usually indicates a comorbidity or another diagnosis.
- **Creatine kinase (CK)**: CK is the most widely used enzyme to diagnose and monitor neuromuscular diseases. The other muscle enzyme tests are for the levels of aldolase and LDH, which are all important when diagnosing ME/CFS and especially FMS in ruling out other muscle pathologies. Aldolase is involved in the breakdown of glucose, fructose and galactose. LDH helps convert lactic acid to pyruvic acid.
- **Cholesterol**: Lipoproteins are combinations of lipids (fats) and proteins that transport cholesterol in the blood. High-density lipoproteins (HDL) transport cholesterol from the tissues of the body to the liver. HDL cholesterol is therefore considered the 'good' cholesterol. The higher the HDL cholesterol level, the lower the risk of coronary artery disease. Low-density lipoprotein (LDL) transports cholesterol from the liver to the tissues of the body. LDL cholesterol is therefore considered the 'bad' cholesterol.
- **ESR**: The erythrocyte sedimentation rate (also known as the SED rate) also measures inflammation in the body but is much cruder than the CRP. It actually measures how fast red blood cells fall to the bottom of a test tube. An ESR is usually high during flare-ups of inflammatory diseases

such as rheumatoid arthritis. As with CRP, it is normally low or normal in ME/CFS and FMS patients.

- **Polymerase chain reaction (PCR)**: This is a universally used technique to rapidly multiply millions of copies from a small DNA sample, allowing scientists to amplify it so it can be analysed much more accurately. It is an extremely versatile test and can use other body fluids as well as blood to screen for bacteria, fungi and parasitic infection as well as viruses (as plenty of people who have had PCR testing for Covid-19 will testify).

- **Triglycerides**: The major form of fat. A triglyceride consists of three molecules of fatty acid combined with a molecule of the alcohol glycerol. The levels if high may indicate an imbalance of free radicals and antioxidants in the body. In 2012 a study showed that ME/CFS patients have higher levels of triglycerides than a control group. The research team concluded this was due to oxidative stress-induced-damage to lipids and proteins.

- **U&Es (urea and electrolyte balance)**: Urea is the major organic component of human urine comprised of broken-down amino acids. A U&E test is commonly used to detect abnormalities in blood chemistry, primarily kidney (renal) function and dehydration.

Hormone tests

In both ME/CFS and FMS the hypothalamus and the pituitary gland are both affected by toxic overload which can lead to many hormonal problems affecting any endocrine (hormone-producing) gland. Tests for the main hormones can identify a problem which may be due to a problem in the central control rather than a disease in the individual endocrine organ. I therefore advise patients who start the Perrin Technique to have a retest periodically to see if the hormonal disturbance has rectified after a course of treatment.

- **Thyroid tests**: There are two main thyroid tests, for triiodothyronine (T3) and for thyroxine (T4). There are three different types of T3 test:

total T3, free T3 and T3 uptake. The two most common blood tests for hypothyroidism in men and women are a T4 blood test and a serum TSH (thyroid stimulating hormone) blood test. A T4 blood test will measure the level of T4 hormones in the blood.

- **Adrenal tests**: By measuring levels of the adrenal hormones cortisol and dehydroepiandrosterone (DHEA) in the saliva one can assess how the body responds to stress. Cortisol levels can be tested at home by taking a saliva sample immediately on waking, and then four further samples throughout the day. The short synacthen test screens for adrenal insufficiency by measuring serum cortisol before and after an injection of synthetic adrenocorticotrophic hormone (ACTH), normally secreted from the anterior pituitary gland.

- **Prolactin** is a single-chain protein hormone closely related to growth hormone. It is secreted by the anterior pituitary gland. It is also synthesised and secreted by a broad range of other cells in the body, most prominently various immune cells, the brain and the decidua (remains) of the pregnant uterus after birth.

- **Follicle stimulating hormone (FSH)** is released by the pituitary gland into the bloodstream and stimulates the growth of ovarian follicles before the release of an egg at ovulation. In men it stimulates sperm production.

- **Luteinising hormone (LH)** is a protein hormone that causes ovulation; it is released by the anterior pituitary gland in women. In men, LH stimulates production of testosterone.

- **Insulin**: This hormone is produced in the pancreas and causes glucose to leave the blood and enter the cells for use as energy or for storage, glucose being the body's main source of energy. Testing for glucose levels is important for establishing whether or not the patient is diabetic. Diabetes is the most common cause of abnormal glucose levels. Too little insulin, or too much, may be a sign of diabetes of which there are two types:
    - Type 1 diabetes is an autoimmune disease that causes the insulin producing beta cells in the pancreas to be destroyed leading to little

Appendix 2

or no insulin at all. It is commonly diagnosed in children; however, the condition can develop at any age.
- With type 2 diabetes, the body still makes insulin but the person develops 'insulin resistance'. This is when cells in your body don't respond well to insulin and can't use glucose for energy leading to more insulin being produced in a vicious circle. Eventually, sugar levels in the blood go up leading to type 2 diabetes.

Liver function tests (LFTs)

Liver enzymes are proteins that help trigger chemical reactions that your body needs to function. Too much or too little of the following enzymes found in the blood may signal a problem with the liver that needs further investigation.

- **Albumin (Alb)** is the main protein produced by the liver found in the blood. It keeps fluid from leaking out of blood vessels; nourishes tissues; and transports hormones and other chemicals through the blood.
- **Alanine transaminase (ALT)** converts alanine, an amino acid found in proteins, into pyruvate, important for several metabolic pathways including energy production. In healthy people ALT levels in the blood are low.
- **Aspartate transaminase (AST)** is found mostly in the liver and muscles and is released into the blood when the liver is damaged. There is a small amount of AST found in healthy blood but higher-than-normal amounts may be a sign of a health problem.
- **Alkaline phosphatase (ALP)** is also found at high levels in bones and varies with age and gender. High levels of ALP are seen in pregnant women and children undergoing growth spurts.
- **Gamma glutamyl transpeptidase (GGT)** helps transport other molecules around the body. It plays a significant part in helping the liver metabolise drugs and other toxins and is affected by alcohol intake. GGT is often measured relative to another enzyme, such as ALP. That is, both

GGT and ALP are raised in liver problems whereas if GGT levels are normal and ALP high, it indicates possible bone disease.
- **Total bilirubin (TBIL)**: Bilirubin is an orange-yellow pigment that occurs when part of your red blood cells are broken down by the liver. It travels through your liver, gallbladder and digestive tract before being excreted. It is used to detect jaundice, anaemia and liver disease but can be naturally high due to a genetic condition, Gilbert's syndrome.

Parasitic infection tests

Some patients with ME/CFS and FMS have been found to suffer from parasitic disorders which need to be tested for as stringently as viral, bacterial or fungal infections. Parasites that could occur alongside or actually lead to ME/CFS or FMS can be nematodes (round worms) or other invading microscopic parasites causing infections that may require further investigation, such as specialised blood tests for Toxoplasma protozoa, Giardia lamblia or Babesia or for nematode infection.

Virology tests

As a viral infection is a common trigger for both ME/CFS and FMS, tests for viral infections are most important in helping understand some of the symptoms of the condition. If one suspects a virus is still active and in the acute phase this will be revealed by an antibody test known as IgM (immunoglobulin M).

It may be that a new virus has recently infected the patient who already has ME/CFS or FMS, aggravating the pre-existing condition and exacerbating symptoms already present. However, if the test shows a positive IgG (immunoglobin G) this detects antibodies from a past infection and is important in identifying the possible viral infection that led to the start or worsening of the symptoms. The IgG test is the antibody test that has become familiar during the Covid-19 pandemic.

Appendix 2

- **Coronavirus-B (Covid-19)**: Coronaviruses (CoV), which thanks to the pandemic of 2020 need no introduction, are a large family of viruses that cause illness ranging from the common cold to more severe diseases. A novel coronavirus (nCoV) is a new strain that has not been previously identified in humans. The novel coronavirus causing severe acute respiratory coronavirus 2 (SARS-CoV-2) was first discovered in China in 2019 and is better known as COVID-19.

- **Cytomegalovirus (CMV) antibody tests**: CMV is a herpes virus that can sometimes cause similar symptoms to EBV. The test detects current active CMV infection IgM, or past CMV infection IgG.

- **Epstein-Barr virus (EBV) test**: Glandular fever, also known as infectious mononucleosis or just 'mono', can be diagnosed with an antibody blood test called a Paul Bunnel test which reacts to blood cells of the sheep, or monospot tests which uses horse's blood to cause the positive test reaction for the Epstein-Barr virus (EBV).

- **Hepatitis**: Most cases of acute hepatitis are due to viral infections: hepatitis B is caused by a hepadna virus; hepatitis C is caused by a flaviviridae virus. Both hepatitis B and C may lead to a chronic form of hepatitis, culminating in liver cirrhosis.

- **Rubella**: The presence of IgM rubella antibodies means a current or recent rubella (German measles) infection. The presence of IgG antibodies confirms immunity against the infection. If the patient has little or no immunity to rubella, the antibody titre result will be 1:8 or less.

Bacteriology tests

One of the main chronic bacterial infections that is being detected in patients with severe ME/CFS and FMS is Lyme disease, also known as borreliosis (page 123). To make a diagnosis of Lyme disease the doctor may take a blood sample. The most common screening tools in clinics worldwide are the ELISA and Western Blot tests which miss many positive cases. However, there are a few private specialised labs that carry out much more accurate tests, such as the Elispot.

Many other bacterial infections can trigger ME/CFS and FMS and a simple blood culture can be done via your family doctor to screen your blood for bacteria or yeasts that might be causing the infection. Gut bacteria play an important part and many studies on ME/CFS and FMS have shown a major disturbance with the microbiome.

Fungal infection tests

Most patients and health practitioners don't even think of testing for mycotoxins yet it was crucial for one of my younger patients who was brought up in a very old house which was full of mould. This teenage boy had a simple urine test at a specialist private lab which detected mycotoxins which were then treated by antifungal and detox regimes. A thorough investigation into fungal infections examines mycotoxins associated with Aspergillus (aflatoxin, ochratoxin and gliotoxin); Penicillium (sterigmatocystin and mycophenolic acid); Tachybotrys (roridin); Fusarium (enniatin and Zearalenone); Chaetomium globosum (chaetoglobosin); and multiple other mould species (ciritin).

Other medical tests: scans and X-rays

Note: both CT and MRI imaging techniques may sometimes deploy the use of chemicals that are injected into the patient before the procedure that enhances the image. This may not be tolerated well in some ME/CFS and FMS patients and so should be discussed with the doctor before any such procedure is carried out.

- **CT scan**: A computerised tomography scan, also known as a CAT scan, uses computers and rotating X-ray machines to create cross-sectional images of all parts of the body. These images provide more detailed information than normal X-ray images and are better at examining bones and joints three-dimensionally than are MRI scans.
- **Echocardiogram**, also known as an 'echo', is a type of ultrasound scan used to examine the heart and nearby blood vessels. A small probe is used to send out high-frequency sound waves that create echoes when

they bounce off different parts of the body. These echoes are picked up by the probe and turned into a moving image on a monitor while the scan is carried out. An echocardiogram may be requested by a heart specialist (cardiologist) or any doctor, including a GP, who thinks there might be a problem with the heart. The test is usually carried out at a hospital or clinic by a cardiologist or a trained specialist called a cardiac physiologist.

- **EEG** or electroencephalogram is a painless test used to find problems related to electrical activity of the brain. Small electrodes are placed on the scalp which then send signals to a computer to record the wave patterns of the brain.
- **ECG** or electrocardiogram checks the heart's rhythm and electrical activity. It is used to investigate symptoms of a possible heart problem, such as chest pain, palpitations, dizziness and shortness of breath, and arrhythmias which all can occur in ME/CFS and FMS.
- **fMRI**: A functional magnetic resonance imaging scan is a type of MRI scan (see below) that is used to measure and map the brain's activity.
- **HRV** or heart rate variability is the variation in the time interval between consecutive heartbeats measured in milliseconds. HRV changes with exercise, hormonal reactions, cognitive processes, plus other metabolic processes and, of course, stress. It can be measured by sophisticated equipment in a hospital setting but can be also monitored with certain strap-on portable devices one can buy online. There are plenty of practitioners world-wide that use HRV for many different disease processes to monitor autonomic disturbance and therefore this may be very useful in monitoring patients with either ME/CFS or FMS.
- **MRI** or magnetic resonance imaging scan uses strong magnetic fields and radio waves to produce detailed images of the inside of the body. It takes longer than the CT scans and makes a much louder noise so is more challenging for many ME/CFS and FMS patients who suffer from hyperacusis. However, it can be more accurate in detecting problems within the brain and nervous system that are hard to see on CT images.
- **PET** or positron emission tomography scan is an imaging technique

that uses a radioactive tracer that can detect the functioning of different internal organs, mainly used to show if the brain is functioning correctly

- **SPECT**, or single photon emission computed tomography scan, is another type of nuclear imaging test looking at the functioning of the brain. It uses a radioactive substance and a special camera to create 3-D pictures. It is excellent in showing blood flow to tissues and organs. Since 2012 dual photon emission computerised tomography has been used in research to image the neuro-lymphatic drainage of cerebrospinal fluid in perivascular and paravascular spaces but the clinical use of these advanced scanning techniques remains rare at the present time (2021).

- **Ultrasound** scans use a small probe to send out high-frequency sound waves that create echoes when they bounce off different parts of the body which are turned into an image on a monitor while the scan is carried out. They are most often used to examine the foetus in pregnancy but can be used to examine the health of most organs in the body.

- **X-rays** are a type of invisible radiation that can pass through the body, being absorbed at different rates by different parts of the body, usually for the examination of bones and joints.

Appendix 3

The Perrin Questionnaire for chronic fatigue syndrome/ME (The PQ-CFS)

The following is the questionnaire (the PQ-CFS) I use as part of the assessment of new ME/CFS and FMS patients. (Note that joint swelling (Question 16) is not a symptom of ME/CFS or FMS. There may be joint pain or swelling in a limb due to oedema but arthritic-type joint swelling means that there is a comorbidity of arthritis, especially if the swelling is in more than one joint, or other conditions causing joint inflammation such as SLE.) The maximum score is therefore 49 for women, 47 for men. Also note that the scores are part of the assessment and do not always reflect the actual severity of the patient's condition but generally <15 = a mild case; 15-25 = average; 25-35 = severe and 35+ = very severe. To make a more accurate prognostic score one should follow the system detailed in Chapter 10 of *The Perrin Technique 2nd Edition* and, better still, see a licensed Perrin Technique practitioner if possible.

Please take your time and make sure you answer all the questions. You do not have to complete the questionnaire all at once, as long as all questions are answered. (Male patients do not answer questions 49 and 50.)

Please tick the box only if the answer to each of the following is yes. Leave blank if the answer is no.

1. I suffer from physical fatigue ☐

2. My concentration is reduced ☐

3. I have difficulty getting to sleep ☐

4. I often have vivid/weird dreams ☐

5. My sleep is usually disturbed ☐

6. I have problems with short-term memory ☐

7. I find it difficult to read ☐

8. I get 'muzziness' in the head/brain fog ☐

9. I suffer from sinusitis ☐

10. I suffer from head pain ☐

11. I suffer from neck pain ☐

12. I suffer from shoulder pain ☐

13. I suffer from upper back pain ☐

14. I suffer from lower back pain ☐

15. I suffer from other joint pain ☐

16. I suffer from joint swelling ☐

17. I suffer from general muscle pain ☐

Appendix 3

18. I often suffer from numbness ☐

19. I often suffer from pins and needles ☐

20. I suffer from redness in the face ☐

21. I suffer from frequent rashes ☐

22. I suffer from dry skin ☐

23. I suffer from frequent spots on my forehead ☐

24. I suffer from frequent spots on my back ☐

25. I suffer from frequent spots on my chest ☐

26. I feel depressed ☐

27. I feel anxious ☐

28. I suffer from panic attacks ☐

29. I am sensitive to bright light ☐

30. I am sensitive to loud noise/suffer from tinnitus ☐

31. My temperature fluctuates ☐

32. I suffer from bad breath ☐

33. I suffer from thrush ☐

34. I have problems with my bowels ☐

35. I have problems with my bladder ☐

36. I am sensitive to smells ☐

37. I have food intolerances/allergies ☐

38. I have lumpy breasts ☐

39. I have tenderness/pain in the chest ☐

40. I am frequently breathless ☐

41. I suffer from palpitations ☐

42. I suffer from sore throats ☐

43. I suffer from nausea ☐

44. I suffer from dry eyes ☐

45. I suffer from dry mouth ☐

46. I sweat a lot ☐

47. I suffer from cold hands/feet ☐

48. I suffer from mood swings ☐

(Then the final two questions are for female patients only)

49. I suffer from PMS ☐

50. My symptoms are worse during periods ☐

Appendix 3

The following supplementary question should always be used together with the PQ-CFS as it screens patients for possible disorders such as clinical depression, anxiety or bipolar who will answer (a) or (b) positively; ME/CFS and FMS patients will answer (c), (d) or (e) positively. If they tick (b) and (d) they may have both depression and ME/CFS. Also remember, this question is investigating if the patient suffers from post-*exertional* malaise (PEM) – not post-*exercise* fatigue. Make sure that the patient understands that they must think about how they feel after pushing themselves physically or mentally. Also, the reaction may take up to three days to surface as reflected in the response to (e). .

Supplementary question

Please tick the box that you feel best describes your symptom picture.

Following exertion do your symptoms:

a. always improve ☐

b. sometimes improve ☐

c. always worsen ☐

d. sometimes worsen ☐

e. sometimes initially improve but worsen within three days ☐

Appendix 4

Useful names and addresses

ME/CFS and FMS organisations

UK

Action for ME
Action for ME is a UK charity working to improve the lives of adults and children with ME. They campaign for more research, better services and treatments.

42 Temple Street, Keynsham

BS31 1EH

Tel: +44(0)117 927 9551

questions@actionforme.org.uk www.afme.org.uk

Association of Young People with ME
The Association of Young People with ME (AYME) is a UK charity that provides support for children and young people aged up to 26 who have ME. AYME also offers help and support to parents, carers and professionals in health, education and social care.

PO Box 5766

Milton Keynes MK10 1AQ

Tel: +44(0)8451 23 23 89

info@ayme.org.uk www.ayme.org.uk

Appendix 4

Fibromyalgia Association UK
FMA UK provides information and support to patients and their families. It also provides medical information for professionals and operates a national helpline. They aim to encourage NHS and other funding sources to fund new research projects; helplines are manned mostly by volunteers most of whom are FMS sufferers themselves.
Studio 3007, Mile End Mill
12 Seedhill Road, Paisley
PA1 1JS
Tel: +44(0)844 826 9022 (not for support calls) www.fmauk.org

FORME (Fund for Osteopathic Research into ME)
FORME is a UK charity dedicated to helping osteopathic research into chronic fatigue syndrome (ME/CFS). It has funded research that has led to the scientific support of the Perrin Technique and aims to support further projects looking into the physical nature of ME/CFS. One of its main aims now is to disseminate the findings of Dr Perrin's ongoing research.
www.forme-cfs.co.uk

ME Association
The ME Association (MEA), founded in 1976, funds and supports research and provides information and support, education and training in the field of ME/CFS. It aims to avoid duplicating the work undertaken by other voluntary and statutory agencies. It has a very useful website with listings of local societies throughout the world.
7 Apollo Office Court, Radclive Road, Gawcott
Bucks MK18 4DF
Tel: +44(0)1280 818963
www.meassociation.org.uk

The 25% ME Group
The 25% ME Group exists to support all who have the severe form of ME and those who care for them. This includes people who are housebound or

bedbound and/or wheelchair users. At present there is no other organisation concerned specifically with the needs of the severely affected. It is a unique, nationwide, community-based voluntary group with two paid members of staff and a number of volunteers – most of whom have ME – providing a range of services. Because of the intensity of the symptoms and disabilities experienced by severe ME sufferers, the organisation seeks to alleviate the isolation which having this illness can cause and encourages: communication between members; participation in the Group at a number of levels; assistance with articles; and information for the newsletter and much more.
21 Church St, Troon KA10 6HT
Tel: +44(0) 1292 318611 – Mon–Fri, 09:00-17:00
Email: enquiry@25megroup.org

ME Research UK (MERGE)
MERGE holds the database on all research into ME since 1956, in archive form. contact@meresearch.org.uk, www.meresearch.org.uk

The Young ME Sufferers Trust (Tymes Trust)
A charity dedicated to children and young people with ME and their families. Their entire team work pro bono and in 2010 they received the Queen's Golden Jubilee Award for Voluntary Service, for pursuing the educational rights and advancing the care of children with ME. They played a major role in producing the children's section of the Dept of Health Report on CFS/ME (2002).
PO Box 4347, Stock, Ingatestone CM4 9TE www.tymestrust.org

AUSTRALIA

Emerge Australia
A national organisation providing information, support and advocacy.
www.emerge.org.au/

CANADA

FM-CFS Canada
Provides information about research, connects fellow sufferers and raises awareness about ME/CFS and FMS.
310-1500 Bank Street, Ottawa, Ontario K1H 1B8 office@fm-cfs.ca
Tel (toll-free): 1-877-437-HOPE (4673)

EUROPE
European ME Alliance
A grouping of European national charities and organisations that actively supports patients and campaigns for funding for biomedical research to provide better treatment. www.euro-me.org/

IRELAND

FibroIreland
FibroIreland has been created for people affected by fibromyalgia. It provides general information to help sufferers understand how fibromyalgia affects them and what they can do to manage it. It also explains where to find further information. https://fibroireland.com/

Irish ME/CFS Association
The Irish ME/CFS Association, through its various activities and awareness campaigns, strives to improve the situation for people with ME/CFS and to give them information to empower themselves. The group, which has been run entirely by volunteers for the last seven years, has approximately 400 members from the estimated 10,000 sufferers in the Republic of Ireland.
PO Box 3075,
Dublin 2, Ireland.
Tel: +353 (0)1 235 0965
info@irishmecfs.org www.irishmecfs.org

Irish ME Trust
The Irish ME Trust was established in 1989 to provide information and a counselling service to those affected with ME as well as targeting individual problems on behalf of sufferers. It aims to create awareness in the general public and the medical profession as to the plight of ME sufferers in Ireland and contribute to quality biomedical research studies.
Carmichael House, North Brunswick Street, Dublin 7.
Ireland
Tel: +353 (0)1 890 200 912
info@imet.ie www.imet.ie/index.html

NEW ZEALAND

The Associated New Zealand ME Society (ANZMES)
ANZMES was established to provide support for and publish and distribute information to groups and individuals suffering from or interested in ME/CFS including their families and carers. It is also to provide a national focus for and to represent individual sufferers and support groups for ME/CFS in New Zealand. It promotes research into the study of ME/CFS, and into its causes and treatments and liaises internationally, keeps abreast of current research and helps educate health professionals about ME/CFS.
PO Box 36 307
Northcote, Auckland 1309, New Zealand www.anzmes.org.nz

SOUTH AFRICA

ME CFS Foundation South Africa
Supports people with ME/CFS, FMS and other comorbidities such as POTS (postural orthostatic tachycardia syndrome).
info@mecfssa.org mecfssafoundation@gmail.com

USA

Centers for Disease Control and Prevention
As the USA's health protection agency, the CDC is a federal agency that

Appendix 4

conducts health promotion, prevention and preparedness activities in the USA with the goal of improving overall public health.
1600 Clifton Road, Atlanta,
GA 30329, USA
Tel: +1-800-CDC-INFO (800-232-4636); TTY: (888) 232-6348

The National CFIDS Foundation
CFIDS is a national non-profit organisation that funds research and provides information, education and support to people who have ME/CFS (NB: CFIDS is a former name for ME in the USA). The Foundation publishes a quarterly newsletter, The National Forum,
103 Aletha Road, Needham
MA 02492
Tel: +1-(781) 449-3535
info@ncf-net.org www.ncf-net.org/

PANDORA
(Patient Alliance for Neuroendocrine-immune Disorders Organization for Research & Advocacy)
PANDORA is a grassroots advocacy organisation that promotes awareness of and research into/ME/CFS, fibromyalgia, Gulf War illnesses (GWI), multiple chemical sensitivities (MCS) and chronic Lyme disease.
PANDORA Org, Inc
3209 Charlesgate Ave, SW, Wyoming
MI 49509
Tel: +1-(231) 360-6830
www.pandoraorg.net/

Solve ME/CFS Initiative (formerly The CFIDS Association of America)
This organisation has a great monthly e-newsletter Research 1st, as well as a print publication, the Chronicle, which comes out three times a year. Both publications contain articles on research developments, public policy and media

reports, personal stories and a wealth of information vital to people living with CFS. Archived issues are available on the website in an easy-to-read digital publishing format. The organisation also offers a free webinar series and has a vibrant social media community, where patients can stay connected and share information with one another.
350 N Glendale Avenue Suite B #368,
Glendale, CA 91206
+1-704-364-0016
SolveCFS@SolveCFS.org http://solvecfs.org/

#MillionsMissing
#MillionsMissing is a global movement originated in the USA powered by #MEAction to raise awareness and fight for recognition, education and research for people living with ME. According to their website, millions are missing from their careers, schools, families and communities because of the disease. Millions of dollars are missing from research and clinical education regarding this disease, and millions of medical providers are missing out on proper training to diagnose and help patients manage this illness. Every year since May 2016 #MillionsMissing has banded together as an international community of patients, caregivers and allies to raise awareness and demand action.
#MEAction
3900 San Fernando Road #1010,
Glendale, CA 91204
https://millionsmissing.meaction.net/

The International Association for CFS/ME (IACFS/ME)
The IACFS/ME is a non-profit international organisation geared towards the professional community which promotes and coordinates the exchange of ideas related to CFS, ME and fibromyalgia (FM) research, patient care and treatment. The IACFS/ME publishes a peer review online journal, the Bulletin of the IACFS/ME. The IACFS/ME holds major international conferences which are attended by Dr Perrin, and many of the leading scientists and doctors in the field of ME/CFS, FMS and related illnesses.

Appendix 4

27 N Wacker Drive Suite 416, Chicago
IL 60606
Tel:+1-(847) 258-7248
Admin@iacfsme.org www.iacfsme.org/

OTHER COUNTRIES

ME/CFS is universal and there are dozens of countries which also have ME/CFS national support groups for patients. They can usually be found by searching on the internet. Alas, there are many more countries where the sufferer does not have any official organisation that recognises the existence of the disease. Hopefully, this book can be used to help lobby the relevant authorities in showing that ME/CFS is a real physical entity and should be taken more seriously.

PROFESSIONAL ORGANISATIONS

OSTEOPATHY

UK

General Osteopathic Council, 176 Tower Bridge Road, London, SE1 3LU
Tel: +44 (0) 207 357 6655
info@osteopathy.org.uk

Australia
Osteopathy Australia Postal Address:

PO Box 5044,
Chatswood West, NSW 1515
Tel: (Toll Free) 1800 467 836 Tel: 02 9410 0099
info@osteopathy.org.au

Ireland
Osteopathic Council of Ireland
Gray Office Park, Galway Retail Park, Headford Road, Galway
H91 WC1P
info@osteopathy.ie* Tel: +353(0)1 6768819

Canada
Canadian Osteopathic Association
McKenzie Professional Centre 209 - 1595 McKenzie Avenue Victoria, British Columbia
V8N 1A4
Tel: +1-250-595-7772
www.osteopathic.ca osteopathic.ca@gmail.com

USA
American Osteopathic Association
The AOA also provides health information to patients and media interested in osteopathic medicine.
142 E Ontario St, Chicago,
IL 60611-2864
Tel: +1-888-626-9262
www.osteopathic.org

Chiropractic

UK
General Chiropractic Council
Park House
186 Kennington Park Rd, London
SE11 4BT
Tel: +44 (0) 20 7713 5155
enquiries@gcc-uk.org

Australia
Australian Chiropractors Association

Level 1 / 75 George Street, Parramatta,
NSW 2150
PO Box 255, Parramatta, NSW 2124
Tel: Toll free - 1800 075 003; Tel: +612 8844 0400

Canada
Canadian Chiropractic Association

186 Spadina Ave. Suite 6, Toronto,
ON M5T 3B2
Tel: +1 (416) 585-7902; Toll-free: 1-877-222-9303
info@chiropractic.ca; membership@chiropractic.ca

Ireland
Chiropractic Association of Ireland

39 Clonard Street, Balbriggan, Co Dublin,
K32 W729
Tel: +353 87 392 4275
caiadmin@chiropractic.ie

USA
The American Chiropractic Association

1701 Clarendon Blvd, Suite 200, Arlington,
VA 22209
Tel: +1-703-276-8800
memberinfo@acatoday.org

Physiotherapy

UK
The Chartered Society of Physiotherapy
14 Bedford Row, London,
WC1R 4ED
Tel: +44 (0)20 7306 6666
enquiries@csp.org.uk

Australia
Australian Physiotherapy Association
Level 1, 1175 Toorak Road, Camberwell,
VIC 3124
PO Box 437 Hawthorn BC VIC 3122
Tel: 1300 306 622 (within Australia); (+61 3) 9092 0888 (international calls)

Canada
Canadian Physiotherapy Association
955 Green Valley Crescent, Suite 270, Ottawa, Ontario,
K2C 3V4
Tel: +1 (613) 564-5454; (800) 387-8679
information@physiotherapy.ca

Ireland
Irish Society of Chartered Physiotherapists
Royal College of Surgeons in Ireland,
St Stephen's Green,
Dublin 2, D02 H903
Tel: +353 1 402 21 48
info@iscp.ie

Appendix 4

USA
The American Physical Therapy Association

111 North Fairfax Street, Alexandria,
Virginia 22314-1488
Tel: +1-800-999-2782
memberservices@apta.org

Afterword

Aisling Wharton: recovered ME/CFS patient

I was 40 years old with two young children when I came down with a cold virus that left me incredibly fatigued. I was a healthy nutrition coach and rarely got sick, used to fighting off a cold with home remedies within 24 hours, but this time was different.

As I pushed my child in the stroller up the street it felt as though I was pushing through a force field. I had a sense this must be CFS, but my GP dismissed it. Subsequently, I began to catch a cold every three months, and after each one I was left more fatigued to the point that everyday tasks became exhausting, and I felt glued to the chair after putting dinner on the table. After a year, I saw an integrative doctor who diagnosed me with ME/CFS, but after a slight improvement I began to go downhill again. When I didn't have help at home or my husband travelled and the physical demands of family life increased, I would be knocked back further each time, going down to 70%, 60%, 50% of normal energy capacity and brain function.

My children were seven and five when I found myself crawling from the bedroom to the kitchen one morning, unable to walk even a few steps. This was my lowest point in my ME/CFS journey, four years after onset. I needed a wheelchair and was at about a 2 out of 10 in the

Afterword

functioning scale. I could not stand up for more than a few minutes. It felt like wading through quicksand when I walked. My husband had to wash my hair, as well as do all the cooking and childcare. Even a phone conversation was exhausting, due to the effort of speaking a little louder. Being in a restaurant became unbearable with all the noise and sensory input being too much for my nervous system. I had brain fog and difficulty finding words or remembering at times.

I continued my years' long search for answers and came across the Perrin Technique through a recovered patient. When I read Dr Perrin's first book it all made sense. I'd had disabling pain problems due to repetitive strain injury from working in the corporate world many years earlier, and the description of how postural disturbance of the thoracic spine can be a causal factor in ME fitted my picture. I also knew my body had difficulty with detoxifying chemicals and toxins, due to genetic factors. Since there were no Perrin practitioners in the US, I made it my mission to bring the Perrin Technique to the States and set up a workshop for practitioners to train with Dr Perrin.

The half rule, doing 50% of your capacity, was a key learning from Dr Perrin. I knew, as a mother it would be difficult to limit my activity and would take longer to recover. I did weekly treatments for six months without seeing any change and began to wonder if it would work for me. I persevered and after eight months I gradually began to feel more energy. I'd used a mobility scooter to get around for years but eventually began walking a few more blocks each week. After three years I was walking around New York City again! As I got back into life it was challenging not to overdo it and I did have some relapses, but I continued with treatment monthly and recovered to the point that I now walk everywhere and delight in hiking with my family. I even began running for the first time in my life. I now enjoy coaching fatigue patients back to health, integrating the many modalities that facilitate recovery.

Aisling Wharton, Integrative Health Coach, NY, USA
www.aislingwharton.com

Index

acne, 82
Action for ME, 146
active head rest, 75
adapted back sculling, 113
adrenal gland
   surgery and, 122
   tests (of function), 134
   see also hypothalamic-pituitary-adrenal axis
aerobic exercise, 115
aetiology (causes) of ME/CFS and FMS, 93–95
air travel, 119
alanine transaminase (ALT), 135
albumin, 135
alcohol, 78, 111, 135
alimentary canal *see* gut
alkaline phosphatase (ALP), 135, 136
alpha waves, 12, 68, 117
Alzheimer's disease, 125
American Chiropractic Association, 155
American College of Rheumatology, 22
American Osteopathic Association, 154
American Physical Therapy Association, 157
amitriptyline, 112
amyloid beta (beta amyloid), 125
ANA (anti-nuclear antibody) test, 130
anaesthetics, 122
   in childbirth, 120
   general, 120, 121
   supplements and, 121

ANF (anti-nuclear factor) test, 130
antibody (immunoglobulin) tests, 130
   viral infection, 136, 137
antidepressants, tricyclic, 112
antimicrobial properties of garlic, 86–87
anti-nuclear antibody (ANA) test, 130
anti-nuclear factor (ANF) test, 130
antiperspirants, 110
Anzymes (Associated New Zealand ME Society), 150
Aselli, Gasparo, 10
aspartate transaminase (AST), 135
assessment of patient
   Perrin Questionnaire for CFS, 141–145
   physical examination, 34, 46, 47, 88, 127
Associated New Zealand ME Society (ANZMES), 150
Association of Young People with ME (AYME), 146
athletes (sportspeople) and thoracic spine, 51
Australia
   professional organisations, 153, 155, 156
   support organisation, 148
autoimmune disease, 29, 130, 134
autonomic nervous system, 11, 31–32, 43, 51
   disturbances/dysfunction, 22, 23, 33, 98, 102
      cold exposure and, 109
      toxins and, 27

see also parasympathetic nervous
    system; sympathetic nervous system
awakening, 106–107
AYME (Association of Young People with
    ME), 146

back massage, 73, 74
back pain, 8
    low, 7, 108
back sculling, adapted, 113
backstroke, 113
bacteriological infection tests, 137–138
Balfour, Dr William, 22
basal ganglia, 60, 78, 81
baths and showers, 107–109
bed
    getting out of, 107
    sleeping position, 77
bedtime, 111–113
bee propolis, 87
Bell, Dr David, 20
Benson, Jade (case), 3–6
benzene, 26
beta amyloid, 125
Big Pharma, 49–50
bilirubin, 136
biofeedback, 11–12, 27
biomechanical disorder, ME/CFS as, 8, 15,
    40–41, 59
biophysical disorder, ME/CFS as, 19, 34,
    52
birth *see* childbirth
blood
    cell counts, 131–132
    circulation, 9
    pressure, and getting out of bed, 107
    tests, 50, 132–133
blood–brain barrier, 11–12, 27
blue light shielding, 117
borreliosis (Lyme disease), 125, 137
bra(s), 110
bradycardia, 96
brain
    cerebrospinal fluid (CSF) and its flow,
        8, 12

    foggy, 96
    lymphatic drainage from *see* lymphatic
        system
    showers and baths and, 107–109
    see also blood–brain barrier *and*
        specific parts of brain
breast
    lymphatic tissue (female versus male),
        102
    massage, 72, 74
    Perrin's Point, 38–43
breastfeeding, 121
breaststroke, 113
Brennan, Noel (case), 90–91

C-reactive protein, 132
C3 and C4 (complement), 130
Caesarean section, 120
calcium measurements, 132
Canada
    professional organisations, 154, 156
    support organisation, 149
carbon monoxide (CO) poisoning, 26,
    124
cardiac *see* heart
Carruthers, Bruce M, 21, 49
cases (author's), 7–8, 37, 123–124
    Jade Benson, 3–6
    Noel Brennan, 90–92
causes of ME/CFS and FMS, 94–96
CBT-I, 111
Centers for Disease Control and
    Prevention (CDC), 150–153
central nervous system (CNS), 12, 94–95
    lymphatic system *see* lymphatic system
    toxin/poison build-up, 13, 28, 33, 53,
        78, 81, 94–95, 104, 122
    see also brain; spinal cord
cerebrospinal fluid (and flow/drainage),
    8–9, 12, 94
    reflux of toxins back into CSF, 33,
        40
cervical effleurage, 57
cervical isometrics, 65–67
CFCs (chlorofluorocarbons), 26

161

Index

CFIDS (chronic fatigue and immune dysfunction syndrome; US former name for ME), 20
CFIDS (US national non-profit research-funding organisation), 151
CFIDS Association of America (former name of Solve ME/CFS Initiative), 151–152
CFS *see* myalgic encephalomyelitis
chairs, 77
Chartered Society of Physiotherapy, 156
chemicals, toxic *see* pollutants; toxins
childbirth, 120
   trauma to baby, 93
children and young people
   assessment/examination, 47, 121
   education *see* education
   parents as source of toxic exposure, 122
   support organisations, 146, 148
   technology and, 117
   toxin susceptibility, 29
chillax and relax, 111
chiropractic organisations, 154–155
chlorofluorocarbons (CFCs), 26
cholesterol, 132
chronic fatigue and immune dysfunction syndrome *see* CFIDS
chronic fatigue syndrome *see* myalgic encephalomyelitis
circulation, blood, 9
clavicles, massaging lymph towards, 53
clothes, putting them on, 110
CMV (cytomegalovirus), 137
coeliac disease, 104
coeliac plexus, tenderness, 43–44
cognitive behavioural therapy for Insomnia (CBT-I), 111
cold or cool showers and baths, 108–109
colds, 80, 81, 86–88
collar bones, massaging lymph towards, 53
commuting, 118–119
comorbidities (multiple conditions), 22–23, 129

PQ-CFS score, 141
complement components C3 and C4, 130
computer and TV screens, 116–117
computerised tomography (CT), 138
concertina and siphon effect, 53
contrast bathing, 54
cool or cold showers and baths, 108–109
coronavirus *see* Covid-19
cortisol levels, 134
cosmetics, 110
Covid-19 (SARS-CoV-2; coronavirus), 47, 137
   long (post-Covid syndrome), 103, 125
   tests, 137
   vaccine, 87
cranial rhythmic impulse (CRI; cranial rhythm; cranio-sacral rhythm; involuntary mechanism; primary respiration), 44, 58
   disturbances, 45
   treatment regarding, 58, 68
cranial techniques, 58, 103
cranio-cervical instability, 64–65
cranio-sacral rhythm *see* cranial rhythmic impulse
cranio-sacral techniques, 47, 59
crawl, front, 114
creatine kinase, 132
Cribb, Julian, 26
cribriform plate, 12, 14, 32
crop spraying, 123
cross-crawl, 64
CT (computerised tomography), 138
cycling, 115–116
cytomegalovirus (CMV), 137

defining ME/CFS, 21–22
dehydroepiandrosterone (DHEA), 134
delta waves, 12, 13, 68, 108
dental fillings, 123
deodorants, 110
depression, 50, 145
detoxification (toxin/poisons removal/ drainage), 9
   genetic ability, 29

Index

liver, 103
    problems (incl. restricted drainage), 14, 25, 127
DHEA (dehydroepiandrosterone), 134
diabetes, 134–135
diagnosis, 19, 50
    author's theory, 1, 7
    by exclusion, 50, 52, 129
    pathological (lab) tests, 50, 129–138
    see also symptoms and signs
diet and nutrition, 77–78
    supplements see supplements
    toxicity and, 28–29
    see also mealtimes
Donaldson, Sir Liam, 21
dorsal rotation exercises, 61, 127
dorsal spine see thoracic spine
dressed, getting, 110
drugs (pharmaceuticals)
    Big Pharma, 49–50
    for sleep problems, 112–113

EBV (Epstein–Barr virus), 137
ECG (electrocardiogram), 139
echinacea, 87
echocardiography, 138–139
education
    returning to, 117–118
    travel to/from place of, 118–119
EEG, 139
effleurage, 57, 58
    lubrication, 53
    for FMS, 55
electrocardiogram (ECG), 139
electroencephalogram (EEG), 139
electrolyte balance, 133
Ellis, Dr Jason, 111
Emerge Australia, 148
employment see work
encephalomyelitis
    meaning, 20
    myalgic see myalgic encephalomyelitis
endometriosis, 97
endomysial antibody, 130
environmental factors (chemicals/pollutants), 25–26, 94, 122–124
ephapses, 39, 44
epigastrium, 43–44
epigenetics, 29
Epstein–Barr virus (EBV), 137
erythrocytes see red blood cells
European ME Alliance, 149
exercise (physical activity), 7, 101, 113–116
    half-rule, 60, 64, 65, 83, 105, 114–115

facial massage, 69, 70, 73, 74
fascia, 44
females see women
FibroIreland, 149
Fibromyalgia Association UK, 148
fibromyalgia syndrome (fibromyalgia/FMS)
    causes, 93–95
    dos and don'ts, 106–113
    FAQs, 93–129
    ME/CFS compared with/similarities to, 22–23, 101–102
    naming/defining/meaning of disease, 20, 22–23
    pathological (lab) tests, 50, 129–138
    patient groups affected by, 102–103
    patient support organisations, 146–152
    post-traumatic, 56
    stages in development, 31–48
    symptoms and signs see symptoms and signs
    toxins and see toxins
    treatment protocal, 55
fictitious illness syndrome, 118
flu, 80, 86–87
flying, 119
FM-CFS Canada, 149
follicle-stimulating hormone (FSH), 134
food see diet and nutrition
FORME (Fund for Osteopathic Research into ME), 147
front crawl, 114
FSH (follicle-stimulating hormone), 134
full blood count, 131–132

Index

functional MRI, 139
Fund for Osteopathic Research into ME (FORME), 147
fungal infection tests, 138

GABA (gamma-aminobutyric acid), 60
gamma-aminobutyric acid (GABA), 60
gamma-glutamyl transpeptidase (GGT), 135–136
garlic, 86–87
Garvey, Sir William, 22
gastrointestinal system *see* gut
gastroparesis, 97
General Chiropractic Council, 154
genetic predisposition/susceptibility
    to illnesses (in general), 25
    to ME/CFS, 93–94, 121, 127
    to posture-related problems, 37
    to toxicity, 29
German measles (rubella), 137
glucose levels, testing, 130
gluten, 28, 77, 104, 110, 130
glymphatic system *see* lymphatic system
graded exercise therapy, 113, 116
grapefruit seed extract, 87
Griesz-Brisson, Dr Margareta, 124
gut (alimentary canal; gastrointestinal system)
    leaky, 28
    microbiome, 28–29, 138
    toxins in, 28–29
    see also gastroparesis; irritable bowel

haematocrit, 131
haemoglobin amounts, 131
hairdresser, 123
half-rule (exercise), 60, 64, 65, 83, 105, 114–115
head massage, 70, 74
head rest, active, 75
health (good), return to, 76–81
heart (cardiac...)
    ECG (electrocardiogram), 139
    rate (and beats per minute), 96
    variability, 139
    rhythm, 39
    ultrasound (echocardiography), 138–139
heavy-metal toxin, 25, 88, 110
hepatitis B and C, 137
hobbies and pastimes, 116
holidays, 119
home (and household), 122–124
    crop spraying and risk to people at, 123
    parents bringing toxins to, 122
    self-help advice/exercises, 59–73
hormesis, 110
hormones, 50–51, 133–135
    biofeedback, 11–12, 27
    hypothalamus and, 11, 27, 102, 112, 133
    sleep and, 112
    tests, 133–135
    women's, 102
hot baths and showers, 108
household *see* home
hydrotherapy, 107–109
hypermobility
    low lumbar region, 50
    spinal joints, 64–67
hypersomnia, 111
hypothalamic-pituitary-adrenal axis and surgery, 121–122
hypothalamus, 11, 13, 27, 51, 94, 102, 133
    bedtime and, 112
    hormones and, 11, 27, 102, 112, 133
    hot climates and, 119
    shower/bath temperature and, 107–108
    sleep–wake cycle and, 106–107
    toxins and, 27

IACFS/ME (International Association for CFS/ME), 152–153
ICD 8 and ICD 10, 19
imaging, 138–139
immune cells counts, 132
immune system, 23, 29, 80–81, 86, 87, 102
    overactive response, 80–81
    supplements and, 80–81

treatment and the, 50, 51
see also neuro-immune system
immunoglobulin tests *see* antibody test
infections, tests for, 137–139
inflammation, reducing, 54
influenza (flu), 80, 86–87
insomnia, 111
insulin, 134–135
International Association for CFS/ME, 152–153
International Consensus Criteria (ICC), 21
International Statistical Classification of Diseases (ICD 8 and ICD 10), 19
involuntary mechanism see cranial rhythmic impulse
Ireland
    professional organisations, 154, 155, 156
    support organisations, 149–150
irritable bowel, 98

jet-lag, 119
jigsaw puzzle analogy, 83–86
job *see* work
joint hypermobility, strengthening exercises, 64–67

Kinmonth, Professor John, 10

lab (pathological) tests, 50, 129–138
labour, 120
Lapp, Dr Charles, 121–122
leaky gut, 28
leptin, 102
LH (luteinising hormone), 134
liver
    alcohol and, 78, 111, 135
    detoxification, 103
    function tests (LFTs), 135–136
locus coeruleus, 108–109
lubrication for effleurage, 58
lumbar spine, strengthening exercises for lower region, 68
luteinising hormone (LH), 134
Lyme disease, 125, 137

lymph, 40, 44
    flow, 53
        breast massage and, 72
        in healthy versus dysfunctional vessels, 41
        retrograde flow, 33, 41, 42
        sluggish flow, 40
lymphatic system (and drainage from CNS; glymphatic system; neurolymphatics), 1, 9, 12, 32–33, 40–41
    flow *see* lymph
    massage aiding drainage *see* massage
    pumping mechanisms *see* pumping mechanism
    sleep and, 12–13
    toxins and poisons and, 30, 93
    varicosities *see* varicose lymphatics

magnesium levels and surgery, 121
magnetic resonance imaging (MRI), 139
    functional (fMRI), 139
male–female comparisons, 102–103
manual approaches/techniques/therapy (incl. manipulation), 57, 61
    osteopathy and, 52
    Perrin Technique incorporating, 15
massage, 53
    self/at-home, 68–75
ME *see* myalgic encephalomyelitis
ME Association (MEA), 147
ME CFS Foundation South Africa, 150
ME Research UK (MERGE), 148
mealtimes, 110–111
    sleep and, 112
mean corpuscular haemoglobin (MCH)
mean corpuscular haemoglobin concentration (MCHC), 131
mechanical disorder, ME/CFS as, 8, 15, 40–41, 59
megalymphatics, 40, 41, 43, 47
melatonin, 107, 113
    jet-lag and, 119
mental activity, 76

165

Index

mental disorder (psychological disorder), doctors viewing ME/CFS as, 34–35
men–women comparisons, 102–103
mercury, 25, 26, 87–88
MERGE (ME Research UK), 148
microbiome (gut), 28–29, 138
mild stream bathing, 109
#Millions Missing, 152
mobile phones (incl. smartphones), 124
    young people/children, 117
monitor and TV screens, 116–117
movement
    healing aided by, 57, 58, 61
    in strengthening exercises, avoiding, 65, 67
MRI *see* magnetic resonance imaging
Munchausen's disease by proxy, 118
musical instrument-playing, 116
myalgic encephalomyelitis (chronic fatigue syndrome/CFS; myalgic encephalomyelitis/ME)
    as biomechanical disorder, 8, 15, 40–41, 59
    as black hole of medicine, 19
    causes, 93–95
    dos and don'ts, 106–113
    FAQs, 93–129
    FMS compared with/similarities to, 22–23, 101–102
    naming and defining of the disease, 20, 21–22
    outlook *see* prognosis and outlook
    pathological (lab) tests, 50, 129–138
    patient groups affected by, 102–103
    patient support organisations, 146–153
    Perrin Questionnaire for, 141–145
    stages in development, 31–48
    symptoms and signs *see* symptoms and signs
    toxins and *see* toxins
    vicious circle leading to, 13–15

nasal release, 69, 73, 74
National CFIDS Foundation, 151, 151
neck massage, 74

back, 73, 74
front, 71, 74
nervous system, 31–32
    autonomic *see* autonomic nervous system; parasympathetic nervous system; sympathetic nervous system
    central *see* central nervous system
    peripheral, 31
    somatic, 31
neuro-immune system, 47
    disorders, 29
neurological disorder, ME/CFS as, 19, 34, 50, 51
neurolymphatic system *see* lymphatic system
neuropeptide P, 60
neurotoxins, 26, 27–28, 110, 116, 128
    children, 122
    effects, 27–28
    pollutants, 25, 26
New Zealand, support organisation, 150
nutrition *see* diet

occupation *see* work
oils for massage, 53, 70
organisations and associations
    professional, 153–157
    support, 146–152
organophosphates, 26, 116
osteochondrosis of spine (Scheuermann's disease), 37
osteopathy, 52–53, 59–60
    organisations, 147, 153–154
outlook *see* prognosis and outlook

packed cell volume, 131
pain, 60
    back *see* back pain
    ME/CFS versus FMS, 101–102
PANDORA, 151
parasitic infection tests, 136
parasympathetic nervous system, 32
parents as source of toxic exposure, 122
pastimes and hobbies, 116

Index

pathogenesis (development) of ME/CFS and FMS, 31–48
pathological (lab) tests, 50, 129–138
pedometer, 115
Perrin Questionnaire for CFS, 141–145
Perrin technique
    10 steps/stages, 57–59
    aftercare, 46
    for conditions other than ME/CFS and FMS, 124–126
    the facts/how it works, 7–15, 103–104
    frequency, 88, 105–106
    jigsaw puzzle analogy, 83–86
    responses, 104
        side effects and initially feeling worse, 81–83
Perrin's Point, 38–43
perspiration problems, 99
pesticides, 26, 116
PET scan, 139–140
pharmaceuticals *see* drugs
physical activity *see* exercise
physical disorder, ME/CFS as, 19, 34, 52
physical examination, 34, 46, 47, 88, 127
physical signs *see* symptoms and signs
physiotherapy organisations, 156–157
phytosterols, 87
pineal gland, 106–107
pituitary gland, 133, 134
    see also hypothalamic-pituitary-adrenal axis
placebo treatments, 81, 104
plant sterols, 87
platelet counts, 131
poisons *see* toxins and poisons
pollutants, 25–26, 94, 122–124
polycystic ovary syndrome, 97
polymerase chain reaction, 133
positron emission tomography scan, 139–140
post-Covid syndrome (long-Covid), 103, 125
post-exercise malaise/fatigue, 101, 113, 145
post-exertional malaise (PEM), 99, 101, 145
post-nasal drip, 100

postural orthostatic tachycardia syndrome (POTS), 107, 150
potassium levels and surgery, 121
pregnancy, 120–121
prevention of ME/CFS and FMS, 127–128
professional organisations, 153–157
prognosis and outlook
    calculating, 89
    initially feeling worse (with Perrin Treatment) and, 82, 104
prolactin, 134
propolis (bee), 87
psychological disorder, doctors viewing ME/CFS as, 34–35
pumping mechanism (lymphatic system), 10, 44–45
    dysfunction, 10, 40, 50
pupil dilation, 46

radiological tests, 138–139
Ramsay, Dr Melvyn, 21
reconditioning, 60, 113, 127
recovery (remission), 103, 124–125
    jigsaw puzzle of, 83–87
    recurrence following, 126–127
    speed, 105
recurrence (relapse), 126–127
red blood cells (erythrocytes; RBCs)
    counts, 131
    sedimentation rate (ESR), 132–133
reflux (lymphatic), 41
    reflux of toxins back into CSF, 33, 40
rehabilitation, 113–116
relapse (recurrence), 126–127
relax and chill, 111
remission *see* recovery
respiration, primary *see* cranial rhythmic impulse
retrograde lymph flow, 33, 41, 42
rheumatoid factor, 130
Riste, Dr Lisa, 61
rubella, 137

SAD light, 107
SARS (severe acute respiratory disease), 125

167

Index

SARS-CoV-2 *see* Covid-19
Scheuermann's disease, 37
school
    returning to, 118
    travelling to/from, 118–119
scoring the patient, 46–47
seasonal affective disorder, 107
selenium, 28
self-help advice, 56–70
severe acute respiratory disease (SARS), 125
severe symptoms and signs, 127
    outlook, 89
    support organisation for people with, 147–148
shoulder (exercises)
    dorsal rotation, 61, 126
    hugging, 62
    rolling, 62–63
showers and baths, 107–109
shrugging exercises, 61–62
signs *see* symptoms and signs
single photon emission computed tomography, 140
skin eruptions, 82
sleep, 12–13, 111–113
    alpha waves, 12, 68, 117
    delta waves, 12, 13, 68, 108
    flying and, 119
    problems, 111–113
    sleeping position, 77
    waking up from, 106–107
    see also bed; bedtime
sleep apnoea, 95, 112
sleeping pills, 112
smartphones *see* mobile phones
solar plexus, tenderness, 43–44
Solve ME/CFS Initiative, 151–152
somatic nervous system, 31
South Africa, support organisation, 150
SPECT, 140
spinal block, 120
spinal cord
    cerebrospinal fluid (CSF) and its flow, 8, 12
    lymphatic drainage from *see* lymphatic system
spine
    dorsal/thoracic *see* thoracic spine
    osteochondrosis (Scheuermann's disease), 37
sportspeople and thoracic spine, 51
sterols, plant, 87
Still, Dr Andrew, 52, 75
stomach emptying, delayed (gastroparesis), 97
strengthening exercises
    hypermobile spinal joints, 64–68
    lower lumbar hypermobility, 68
stress, 51
    avoiding, 77
stretch marks, 45
striae, 45
sub-occipital hypermobility, 64–65, 64–65
substance P (neuropeptide P), 60
supplements (dietary), 78, 78–81, 83, 86–87
    surgery and, 122
    undesired sife effects and excessive use, 79–80
support organisations, 146–152
surgery, 121–122
    supplements and anaesthesia and, 122
Sutherland, William Garner, 44, 52–53
sweating (perspiration) problems, 99
swimming, 113–115
sympathetic nervous system, 4, 10, 11, 18, 31–32, 39
    blackout and, 18
    cold exposure and, 109
    disturbances/dysfunction, 11, 15, 18, 20, 23, 33, 35, 40, 94–95
    pupil dilation due to, 46
symptoms and signs, 33–46, 95–101
    case, 8
    as diagnostic criteria, 20, 22
    early, examining patients for, 128
    outlook calculation and, 89
    in Perrin Questionnaire for, 141–145
    severe *see* severe symptoms and signs
T3 (triiodothyronine), 133–134

T4 (thyroxine), 133–134
technology, 116–117
television (TV) and monitor screens, 116–117
thalamus, 60, 78, 81
thimerosal, 87–88
thoracic duct, 10, 12, 39, 40, 44
　pump, 39, 44–45
　　dysfunction, 10, 40
thoracic rotation (dorsal rotation) exercises, 61, 126
thoracic spine (dorsal spine; upper back), 8, 11, 36–38, 76
　problems, 7, 8, 36–38
　　sport and, 51
　　treatments addressing, 57, 61, 62, 73
　sportspersons and, 51
thyroid tests, 133–134
thyroxine (T4), 133–134
toxins and poisons, 13–15, 25–30
　breastfeeding and, 121
　build-up, 10, 13–15, 28–29, 102
　　in CNS, 13, 28, 33, 53, 78, 81, 94–95, 104, 122
　environmental, 25–26, 94, 122–124
　feeling worse (in Perrin Technique) and, 81–82
　hobbies and, 116
　lymphatic system and, 30, 94
　ME/CFS compared with FMS, 101–102
　neurological *see* neurotoxins
　reflux back into CSF, 33, 40
　removal/drainage *see* detoxification
trace elements, 28
treatment (in general or non-Perrin), 7
　author's theory, 1, 7
　magic bullet, 49–52
　self-help, 59–73
　see also recovery
tricyclic antidepressants, 112
triglycerides, 133
triiodothyronine (T3), 133–134
trophic changes (thoracic spine), 38
TV and monitor screens, 116–117

25% ME Group, 147–148
Tymes Trust, 148

ultrasound, 139
　cardiac (echocardiography), 138–139
United Kingdom (UK)
　professional organisations, 153, 154, 156
　support organisations, 146–148
United States (USA)
　professional organisations, 154, 155, 157
　support organisation, 150–153
university, 118
urea and electrolyte balance, 133
USA *see* United States

vacations, 119
vaccines, 51
　Covid, 87
　flu, 87–88
Vallex, François, 22
varicose lymphatics, 38–43, 53
　large/huge (megalymphatics), 40, 41, 43, 47
Verghese, Dr Abraham, 33
viral infection tests, 136–137
vitamin B complex and C, 78–79

waking up, 106–107
walking, 115
Wharton, Aisling 158
white blood cell counts, 131
WHO (World Health Organization), 19, 34
women (females)
　bras, 110
　comparisons with men, 102–103
　pregnancy, 120–121
work (occupation/job/employment)
　returning, 117
　stopping or reducing workload, 76
　toxins in the workplace, 122, 123
World Health Organization (WHO), 19, 34

X-ray imaging, 140

young people *see* children and young people

The Perrin Clinic™

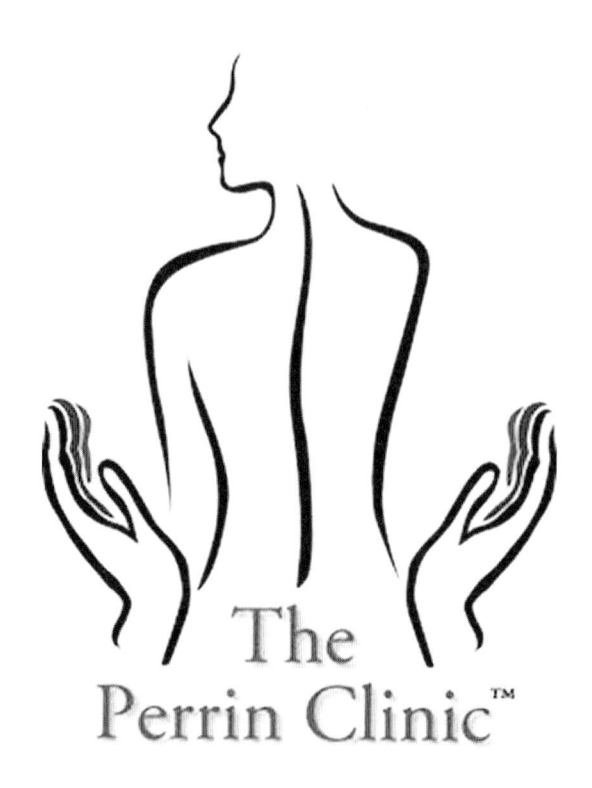

The Perrin Clinic is dedicated to helping all those with ME/CFS, FMS and other related disorders using The Perrin Technique™

The Perrin Clinic is also committed to training and monitoring practitioners who have been licensed to treat patients with The Perrin Technique™

Only licensed practitioners may use the The Perrin Technique™ name and logo as shown below:

The Perrin Technique™

To find your nearest licensed practitioner visit:

www.theperrintechnique.com